Th

10

commandments

of

losing weight

ARLENE NORMAND

Penguin Books

PENGUIN BOOKS
Published by the Penguin Group
Penguin Group (Australia)
250 Camberwell Road, Camberwell, Victoria 3124, Australia
(a division of Pearson Australia Group Pty Ltd)
Penguin Group (USA) Inc.
375 Hudson Street, New York, New York 10014, USA
Penguin Group (Canada)
90 Eglinton Avenue East, Suite 700, Toronto, ON M4P 2Y3, Canada
(a division of Pearson Penguin Canada Inc.)
Penguin Books Ltd
80 Strand, London WC2R 0RL, England
Penguin Ireland
25 St Stephen's Green, Dublin 2, Ireland
(a division of Penguin Books Ltd)
Penguin Books India Pvt Ltd
11 Community Centre, Panchsheel Park, New Delhi – 110 017, India
Penguin Group (NZ)
Cnr Airborne and Rosedale Roads, Albany, Auckland, New Zealand
(a division of Pearson New Zealand Ltd)
Penguin Books (South Africa) (Pty) Ltd
24 Sturdee Avenue, Rosebank, Johannesburg 2196, South Africa

Penguin Books Ltd, Registered Offices: 80 Strand, London WC2R 0RL, England

First published by Penguin Group (Australia), a division of Pearson Australia Group Pty Ltd, 2005

10 9 8 7 6 5 4 3 2

The author and publisher would like to thank Megan Gressor for her valuable assistance in writing this book.

Internal design by Lynn Twelftree © Penguin Group (Australia)
Cover design by Adam Laszczuk © Penguin Group (Australia)
Cover photograph by Monica Telle/photolibrary.com
Author photograph by Rob Homer/Fairfax photos
Typeset in 11/16 pt Bell Gothic by Post Pre-press Group, Brisbane, Queensland
Printed in Australia by McPhersons's Printing Group, Maryborough, Victoria

National Library of Australia
Cataloguing-in-Publication data:

Normand, Arlene.
The 10 commandments of losing weight.

Includes index.
ISBN 0 14 300321 6.

1. Weight loss. I. Title.

613.712

www.penguin.com.au

Contents

*I would like to dedicate this book to my special
and supportive mother; my sons, Jason and
Darren; and my partner, Fred*

*I would like to thank Megan Gressor,
Barbara Northwood, Claire de Medici and Clare Forster
for their assistance*

CHAPTER 1

The lean, mean diet queen

Do you know what they call me? The lean, mean diet queen. I have a reputation for being forthright and firm, and for getting results. I've helped many people overcome weight problems over the years, and I've written this book to help you now.

I'm Arlene Normand, a dietician with a very busy Sydney practice. Over the last decade I've helped thousands of people control their eating problems and I've reached even more through my writing – including my weekly columns in *NW* magazine and the *Wentworth Courier* – and my television and radio work. Every week I receive dozens of letters and emails from people seeking help. So I've had a lot to do with weight issues, and I know the grief they can cause you when you feel you have lost control of your eating.

Many overweight people consider me their dietician of last resort. They come to me when they've tried everything else to lose weight. Often their confidence is at rock bottom. How do I restore their belief that they can lose weight?

I take a holistic approach: I look at the entirety of their life, not just at what they put in their mouth. I don't look at diet in terms of just *what* you eat, but *why* and *when* you eat. There are many reasons for eating beyond mere hunger. Overeating is most often a habit. You may eat because you see food, because you're tired, because you're stressed, because you're unhappy or happy or because you're at a social event. If you don't look at *why* you're eating and address these issues, you'll never win the battle.

It's easy to prey upon the vulnerabilities of people with weight problems. There are countless fad 'diets' and diet products promising weight loss; it's quite a moneymaking racket. So many diet books and magazines promote a totally unhealthy approach to weight loss. Fad diets are based on gimmicks and quick fixes, and advertisements for bogus weight-loss products – creams, patches, non-prescription drugs and dietary supplements – are limitless. But there are no quick fixes to weight problems. These diets are selling hope, and it works – at least in terms of selling books and gimmicks. Have you ever heard or read one of the following promises?

- You'll lose 1 kilogram or more per week for a month or longer without exercising or eating less.
- You'll achieve substantial weight loss, no matter what or how much you eat.
- You'll achieve permanent weight loss even after you stop using the product or following the diet.
- Everyone who uses this product or follows this diet will achieve substantial weight loss.

- You'll achieve substantial weight loss by wearing it on your body or rubbing it into your skin.

The bottom line? There is no miracle solution. You must make lifestyle changes and alter your eating patterns and exercise habits. This is what my book is all about. I was inspired to become a dietician by my own eating problem and an interest in good nutrition, not from a desire to make money. My practice took off because my business is my passion, as well as my vocation – I'm very fortunate because I love what I do!

Weight loss is an area that can be rife with denial and self-delusion. Some people consult a dietician for help with weight loss because they require guidance. Others make the dietician responsible for their own success or failure, and blame the dietician when things go wrong. I believe in making people responsible for themselves. They come to me in the belief that because I've been successful with so many people, I'll be successful with them. So I have to inform them that it doesn't work like that: THEY have to do the work and be accountable for their actions. I'll be there all the way, I'll show them how to achieve their goals, but they've got to make the effort and stay focused. We will work through the issues underlying their eating together, but they are responsible for their own long-term success.

I never let people give up, because I know first-hand the benefits of gaining control of your eating. It really does affect your whole life and equilibrium. When you're binge-ing, you feel out of control. People who eat frenetically become frenetic. I know myself: I've been a chocoholic in my time, and when I ate chocolate it became a compulsive act that I did not even find pleasurable. This kind of compulsion made me feel awful. People who overeat usually don't realise how it affects their mood until they lose weight and feel more in control of their eating and exercise; they notice how their mood has improved. You should always feel your best! When you go shopping for clothes and can purchase whatever you want because everything looks good, you feel great and project a better, more confident self-image. When you're in a healthier frame of mind, you're better able to cope with life – your family, your job, everything. It's a whole new cycle.

I understand this. I've been there. I know what it's like. I've had food issues in the past; controlling my food intake and exercise still makes up an important part of my life. As I was growing up in South Africa I always danced, from the age of about three. We would dance for three or four hours a day, and with so much exercise I was a skinny kid. But from the age of about twelve, as I started maturing I began filling out. It was just normal development, but as dancers we were encouraged to be very slim. This began the dieting that consumed the next decade or so of my life.

I tried just about every diet. The Beverly Hills Diet. The Hip and Thigh Diet. The Gram Diet. The Apple Diet. I've even been on a licorice and prune diet – that was after I went on a trip to the Middle East at age fifteen and put on a lot of weight after eating an abundance of herrings, falafel, nuts, cheese and delicious thick porridge. When I returned, I ate nothing but licorice and prunes in order to get diarrhoea in the hope of losing the weight I'd gained!

For a while I went annually to a health farm where they'd put me on a stringent all-fruit diet, and I'd drop 3 or 4 kilograms in a week. Then I'd go home and put it on again. I'd then go on a fruit diet myself, lose it, put it on again, all the time yo-yoing up and down. Continually starving and bingeing like this is not good for you, but this is how a lot of people live. This is how I used to live. Even when I had children I was always on a diet; I was never content with my body.

When I was seventeen I gave up dancing and went to university. I studied science, and worked with computers, which I enjoyed, but my real interest was always in dietetics. I came to Australia over seventeen years ago, and the opportunity finally arrived to do my Masters degree in nutrition and dietetics. That was when I began to fully realise that the way I had been eating wasn't healthy or normal. I remember looking at one of the dieticians teaching us and thinking, 'She's just eating a sandwich for lunch. How can she look so satisfied just with that?' I'd have a sandwich for lunch and then in the afternoon I'd wonder whether or not to have a Mars Bar. And inevitably, if I had a Mars Bar, I wouldn't stop there – I'd have a Flake, a Crunchie and other sweets. Yet my teacher looked perfectly content with just the sandwich. How I yearned to be 'normal' like her.

That was the start of my regaining control, but it wasn't until I opened my own dietetic practice that I really started to normalise my eating. Hearing other people's stories helped me put my own life into perspective. Clients would tell me about things they'd done, and I'd think, 'I've done that too.' When I helped my clients work out solutions for their problems, I was also working out solutions for myself. And finally I started to live those solutions.

In a way, my yo-yo dieting has actually helped me in my career as a dietician. I think you can only really help people if you have experienced the issues yourself. My clients will often tell me things, such as they've just eaten three packets of Tim Tams and the only way they could stop themselves eating was by taking a sleeping tablet and going to bed. A person who has never binged might think this was mad. But, if you've done it yourself, you can identify with them and explain how you dealt with the issue to help them overcome it themselves.

When I explain to clients what they need to do to take control of their eating, I'm not asking them to do anything I haven't done myself. There is no denying that it takes commitment and perseverance. Even today I still watch my weight. I'll never go a day without thinking about what I'm eating and when I can schedule my exercise. I focus on the consequences of overeating. If I don't feel in control of my eating and exercise, my whole life reflects this. I don't like the way my mood changes after I've eaten too much; I want to be in charge!

I've been in private practice for eleven years; and eleven years ago was when I finally normalised my eating. That was the point at which I achieved my twin goals: to take charge of my own eating and life, and to help other people do the same. I love seeing people regain control of their weight and balance their life. Life balance has to come first, otherwise the weight loss won't happen. If you have a balanced life, you will also have balanced eating. Your eating problem is a sign that you have something uncontrolled in your life — are you bored, tired or stressed? Issues such as these, coupled with your eating problem, can lead to more all-encompassing problems including depression, marriage breakdown or problems with children, which in turn can drive you to eat more. You need balance, and you must take time to focus on the whole you: your mind, your sense of humour, your personality, your skills, your interests. Your external shape is not the only part of you.

My guess is, if you've picked up this book and read this far, you have some issues about weight. Maybe you feel helpless to do anything about it. Perhaps, like some of my clients, you've tried everything else and failed. I know you can succeed! Your life *will* change, but you need to read the entire book before this change can begin. I'm behind you 100 per cent, because I know from personal experience the benefits of taking control of your eating and your life.

In this book, I've presented some of the solutions that have helped my clients (and me) over the last decade. The eating plan I am going to explain to you is simple, practical and easy to live with. You don't have to go out of your way to buy special, expensive food. While you'll almost certainly be eating less than you are now, you won't feel deprived, because it allows you six meals a day, as well as regular treats. Nothing is off limits, as long as you plan for it. It works anywhere, whether you are eating at home, out in a restaurant or at a friend's house. There is no counting this or calculating that, no special foods or unappetising supplements. My plan allows you to enjoy your food as part of a balanced lifestyle, which includes healthy amounts of food, exercise, sleep, work, relaxation and recreation. If there is only one message that you take away from this book, I'd like it to be this: restore balance to your life and you'll not only feel happier and healthier, you'll be able to get your eating under control.

I know my program works because I've done it myself, and so have hundreds of my clients. In fact, some of them have shared their stories to show you that it *can* be done. It is not complicated. In fact, it can be boiled down to ten simple rules, which I've called my 10 commandments.

1
A LIFESTYLE, NOT A DIET
This isn't a short-term fix; it's a way of life.

2
GET ORGANISED
Structure your life and you'll structure your eating.

3
EAT SMALL
Portion control is crucial to losing weight.

4
LEARN TO LEAVE FOOD ON YOUR PLATE
This helps you take control over compulsive eating.

5
NEVER FEEL DEPRIVED
This only encourages bingeing.

6
MAKE A MEAL OF IT
Make a ceremony out of every meal, so that you really
appreciate what you've eaten.

7
EAT SLOWLY
That way, you'll feel satisfied before you've eaten too much.

8
ENJOY YOUR FOOD
It's one of life's great pleasures, not a punishment.

9
MOVE IT!
Exercise is an essential part of losing weight.

10
BALANCE YOUR LIFE
This is a fundamental step in regaining control over
your eating.

There is a bit more to it than that, as you are about to find out, but keep these simple rules in mind and you will be taking the first steps on your way towards a new, healthy and balanced life.

What about kids?

This book is for adults, but what about kids? Childhood obesity is reaching epidemic proportions, principally due to decreased activity, increased consumption of junk food and larger portion sizes. If you think your child is overweight or obese, consult your doctor or dietician for advice. Weight is generally a vulnerable issue for children, so you must handle the matter with sensitivity and caution. Try not to focus on your child's size, because you may encourage low self-esteem and attitudes that can lead to eating disorders. Focus on keeping your child's weight stable while they grow. At the same time, encourage physical activity (start by encouraging a walk to school, sport, and walking instead of driving them everywhere!). Cook the correct portions and leave temptations out of the house, without being obsessive. Childhood obesity is beyond the scope of this book, so seek expert advice if you are concerned.

CHAPTER 2

What are you putting in your mouth?

Why has excess weight become such a serious problem? Why do so many people find it difficult to maintain a healthy weight – or lose a few excess kilos – while maintaining a realistic lifestyle: eating out, socialising, cooking delicious meals, enjoying holidays and coping with stress or fatigue? Over the past twenty years, obesity has increased to epidemic proportions in Australia – we are now officially the second-fattest nation after the United States, and we are getting fatter. Almost half of the Australian population is heavier than it should be. This is shocking news. Are you part of this statistic? If so, you'll know first-hand how terrible the excess weight makes you feel and look – and it has serious consequences on your health.

The causes of this increase in obesity are complex – the high availability of high-kilojoule food, an increase in portion sizes and declining activity levels. We are eating more than we need (or at least differently) and moving less than we should; driving to a takeaway for a high-fat fast-food meal instead of walking to the market to purchase the ingredients for a balanced home-cooked meal.

There has been considerable research into the link between genetics and obesity. Although researchers found a defect gene in experimental mice that appears to influence hunger levels and obesity, they also found that the human body contains a range of genes and chemicals that control appetite. Genetics alone cannot account for the rapid increase in obesity over the past two decades, because this is too short a time to allow for much change in the gene pool. It can only be explained by behavioural factors – changes in our eating and exercise patterns.

DO YOU HAVE A WEIGHT PROBLEM?

Are you overweight? One method of determining whether you are at a healthy weight is by using the Body Mass Index (BMI). Body mass index is calculated by the following formula*.

BMI = weight (in kilograms) ÷ height (in metres) squared

For example, if you weigh 70 kilograms and are 1.7 metres tall:

$$70 \div 1.7^2 = 24$$

According to the Body Mass Index categories (see over the page), you would fall within the high level of the normal range. (*These BMI ranges apply to adults and are not applicable to children under 18.)

BMI categories

Under 18.5	=	underweight
18.5 to 24.9	=	normal range
25 to 29.9	=	overweight
30 to 40	=	obese
Over 40	=	morbidly (dangerously) obese

A healthy weight range equates to a BMI between 18.5 and 24.9. The reason for this range is because your height is not the only factor to consider when establishing your optimum weight. Your bone structure and body shape – you could be an endomorph (muscular, heavy boned and solid), meso-morph (medium build) or an ectomorph (fine-boned with a slight build) – must be taken into account.

Your build is genetically determined. You must be realistic; if you are big boned and/or muscular, you are likely to weigh closer to the upper end of the range. This does not mean that you are fat, merely that you have a more solid build.

MEASURING UP

Another way to check whether you are a healthy size is to measure your waist circumference as a check on your abdominal fat. If you have a waist measurement of 94 centimetres+ (men) or 80 centimetres+ (for women) you are at an increased risk of developing problems such as heart disease and diabetes due to excess abdominal fat. (I will discuss abdominal fat in greater detail in Chapter 14.)

GOOD FOODS, BAD FOODS

Why are you overweight? Do you know exactly what your body has been up to lately, or have you read, seen and heard so much conflicting information about which foods make you fat that you don't know what to believe?

Weight loss is not easy or simple. Food cannot simply be divided into 'good' and 'bad' categories – items that you should and should not eat. Adopting that attitude results in self-denial, and often subsequent bingeing on those foods you have been denying yourself because you believe they are bad – if you think they are forbidden you will want them even more.

Fruit, vegetables, fish, dairy products, eggs and chicken are commonly thought of as 'good' foods; while hot chips, crisps, chocolates, cakes, biscuits, lollies and baked foods are usually considered to be 'bad' foods. (Interestingly, alcohol is often not considered 'bad', and is more accepted as part of a balanced diet, but many people do not realise how loaded it is with 'empty' – meaning no nutritional value – kilojoules.)

You expect to put on weight when you eat 'bad' food, but not when you eat 'good' food, regardless of the quantity. For example, people often eat excess fruit, and cannot understand why they are gaining weight – good food should not be fattening! The important thing to know is that it is the total number of kilojoules you consume on a daily basis, not any one particular food item that determines whether you put on weight.

> ## What is a kilojoule?
>
> A kilojoule is a measure of energy. The number of kilojoules in a food is the gauge of how many energy units that food supplies. The more kilojoule-dense (high in kilojoules) a food, the more energy that food provides. Kilojoules are required to fuel all the body's functions and activities, from basic metabolic tasks such as the heart beating, digestive processes or growing nails and hair, to thinking and walking. The different classes of food supply different amounts of energy: protein supplies 17 kilojoules per gram, carbohydrate supplies 17 kilojoules per gram, alcohol supplies 29 kilojoules per gram and fats supply 37 kilojoules per gram. (Note: 1 calorie = 4.2 kilojoules.)

THE WEIGHT-LOSS EQUATION

The weight-loss equation is simple:

energy in (kilojoules) − energy out (activity and metabolism)
= gain/loss of body weight

If you consume more kilojoules than your body uses in its activities, you will gain weight. Conversely, if you consume fewer kilojoules than your body requires to meet its energy expenditure, you will lose weight.

The weight you gain from excess kilojoules does not depend on the source, whether it be fat, carbohydrates, protein or alcohol. You will, however, gain *more* weight when you consume too much fat, because 1 gram of fat contains more than twice as many kilojoules as 1 gram of protein or carbohydrate. You will be astonished by the quantity of fat hidden in your favourite foods. For example, vegetable quiche is often considered a healthy choice due to the vegetables, but there is an abundance of fat in a quiche – think of the eggs, cheese and cream used in your favourite recipe.

Australians are getting fatter because they have increased their intake of kilojoules while reducing their exercise levels. Many of the excess kilojoules come from soft drinks (which have no fat but are loaded with sugar), lollies, chocolates, biscuits, cakes, deep-fried food, high-carbohydrate muffins, bagels, pretzels and reduced-fat chips. Additionally, portion sizes have grown remarkably and are now accepted as normal, so not only are we eating more high-fat foods, our serves are huge.

THE BLACKLIST

Never blacklist individual foods or entire food groups from your diet, unless you have a food intolerance or allergy. Forget fad diets that omit certain groups such as carbohydrates, dairy or perhaps wheat because the diet maestros claim they are responsible for weight gain. The most important part of successful weight loss is balance, and when you eliminate an entire food group, your body misses out on important nutrients. Moreover, you are likely to feel deprived, increasing the risk of bingeing (more on this topic in Chapter 9).

You can eat everything you enjoy, provided you moderate your choices and keep your portions small. Weight control should not be your only concern when making food choices; it is imperative to enjoy a wide variety of foods to optimise your intake of nutrients. You should not pay more attention to the type of food but to the relative quantities you consume. A meat pie or a doughnut would not be an ideal choice to eat daily, but it is acceptable as an occasional treat. The Healthy Food Pyramid (see below) illustrates the wiser food choices to make, while always being aware of portion size.

THE HEALTHY FOOD PYRAMID

Eat least
Sugar, butter,
margarine, oil, alcohol.

Eat moderately
Protein foods such as lean meat,
fish, poultry, eggs, nuts, seeds, low-fat
dairy products (milk, cheese, yoghurt).

Eat most
Carbohydrate foods such as fruit, vegetables, breads,
cereals, pasta, grains, rice.

Battling the binge

Question: I am a horrific binge eater. When I start eating, I just cannot stop. I end up eating things I do not even like, gorging myself until I feel sick. At the end of each binge I make up my mind never to binge again, but then something upsets me and I am out of control again. I am desperate for help because I cannot live my whole life like this!

Answer: Binge eating is driven by depression, anger and anxiety. It is a psychological disorder that usually has deep roots. Bingeing is a cycle: you feel emotional so you binge, then you feel guilty so you binge again. Stringent dieting can trigger bingeing: there is a tendency to gorge on the foods you feel you are missing. Here are a few tips to help you.

- Stop before the binge escalates – have a bath, go for a walk, do anything that removes you from the source of food.
- Wait – whenever you feel the urge to binge, try to figure out why you are upset and what you can do to overcome these feelings.
- Ask for help. Bingeing usually occurs when you are alone. Visit a friend or phone someone you trust when you feel you are losing control.
- Forgive yourself. Your bingeing has probably been occurring for a long time, so you cannot expect it to stop overnight. Try to make gradual changes to your life, and you are more likely to succeed in ending your tendency to binge.
- If you really cannot stop, seek the help of a professional trained in eating disorders.

Protein

Protein-rich foods build and nourish blood, skin, bones and muscles. They increase the satiety of a meal (satisfying you and keeping hunger pangs at bay). Certain protein foods are high in saturated fat, so the low-fat and lean options are a healthier choice.

Choose: eggs, low-fat yoghurt, low-fat cheese, low-fat milk, peanut butter, nuts, lean meat, skin-free poultry, legumes, low-fat soy products and seeds.

Forget: marbled (fatty) meat, full-fat dairy foods and processed meats such as salami, bologna, pepperoni and bacon.

Carbohydrate

Carbohydrates provide the body with fuel. Protein and fat can also provide the body with energy, but the body prefers carbohydrates. Carbohydrates are classified into two major groups: simple and complex.

Simple carbohydrates are broken down more quickly into their simpler components and absorbed quickly into the bloodstream. They are naturally present in foods such as fruit, vegetables and milk, accompanied by vitamins, minerals and other nutrients. They are also present in less-nutritious foods such as soft drinks and lollies.

Complex carbohydrates – occurring in unrefined whole foods such as brown rice and wholegrain bread – are rich in vitamins, minerals and fibre, and are filling and satisfying.

They are structurally more complex than simple carbohydrates and take longer to be broken down and for the glucose to pass into the bloodstream, which helps stabilise your blood sugar levels. Many foods, particularly fruit and vegetables, contain both simple and complex carbohydrates.

Approximately 60 per cent of your daily kilojoule intake should come from carbohydrate-rich foods – 50 per cent should be made up of complex carbohydrates; the less-processed the better. If you consume too many simple carbohydrates, you may experience highs and lows in blood sugar levels, which cause energy and mood swings.

Choose: wholegrain cereals and breads, wholegrain crackers, whole-wheat pasta, brown rice, legumes, vegetables, salads and fruit.

Enjoy in small portions: chips, cakes, biscuits, doughnuts, pastries, lollies, chocolates and soft drinks.

What is fibre?

Dietary fibre is found in plant foods – cereals (such as corn, oats, wheat and rice), fruit, vegetables, nuts and legumes. Fibre-rich foods require more chewing, which ensures you eat more slowly. They also help you feel satisfied on fewer kilojoules, they reduce hunger and help keep your weight under control. Fibre-rich foods can help regulate blood glucose levels. There are two major categories of fibre: soluble and insoluble.

Soluble fibre is found mostly in oats, psyllium, barley, vegetables, lentils, beans and fruit. Soluble fibre slows the rate of digestion and absorption of food, and is thought to reduce LDL (bad) cholesterol, decreasing your risk of heart disease.

Insoluble fibre is found mostly in wheat bran, wheat-based cereals and pasta, and wholemeal bread. Insoluble fibre keeps your bowels regular, providing bulk to the stool and speeding transit of material through the bowel. It reduces the risk of bowel cancer and other bowel diseases.

Adults should consume approximately 20–30 grams of fibre each day and eat a variety of plant foods.

Here is an example of how to fulfil your daily fibre needs.

Meal	Food	Fibre (g)
Breakfast	30 g All Bran	8.60
	½ cup milk	
Morning tea	1 medium apple (with skin)	3.40
Lunch	2 slices soy linseed bread	9.60
	1 slice cheese	
	¼ cup bean sprouts	0.75
	1 lettuce leaf	0.80
	½ carrot, grated	1.20
Afternoon tea	1 medium banana	3.30
Dinner	grilled fish	
	½ cup peas	4.60
	1 corn cob	4.00
	1 cup mixed salad	2.50
Supper	1 medium pear	3.00
TOTAL		41.75 g

Sugar, fat and alcohol

Go easy on sugar, fat and alcohol, which are at the apex of the Healthy Eating Pyramid. They are concentrated kilojoules with low nutritional value. The exception must be made for the 'healthy' omega-3 fatty acids found in fish oils, canola, flaxseed oil and linseed oil, which are wonderful for your heart and blood.

Save processed sugar, fat and alcohol for occasional treats or special occasions. This includes sugary items such as honey, marmalade, jam, chutney, syrups, sweetened canned fruit, jellies, ice-cream, soft drinks, milkshakes and milk flavourings; and fatty items such as mayonnaise, dripping, creamy soups, gravies and sauces, potato chips and vegetables fried or baked in fat. These are acceptable to consume occasionally in small doses.

Alcohol is extremely high in kilojoules. A standard drink has 8–10 grams of alcohol – and each is an empty kilojoule. When you drink in excess you tend to lose your resolve, which has deleterious effects on weight control. (See page 164 for more about this.)

Dairy

Dairy foods – cheese, yoghurt and milk – are a rich source of calcium, which is necessary for strong bones. Dairy foods ward off high blood pressure, reduce PMS symptoms and lower the risk of bowel cancer. Eating calcium-rich dairy speeds weight loss and helps keep the kilos off! Opt for low-fat milk, yoghurt and cheese. Cheese is high in saturated fat, but a small portion does provide a lot of calcium. Select hard cheeses such as Parmesan and extra-sharp cheddar, which offer more calcium per 30 grams than the softer ones. The eating plan I have created in the next chapter provides for 2 cups of low-fat milk daily, ensuring you are satisfying your recommended daily intake of calcium. If you do not like or cannot tolerate milk, you will need either a calcium supplement or calcium-fortified soya products.

Fat

Of all types of food, fat would have to be the most misunderstood. Once upon a time, all fat was the enemy. Eating as little as possible would supposedly keep you trim. Now, health authorities advocate certain fats as essential for a healthy diet.

Fat is necessary for the absorption of vitamins A, D, E and K through the walls of your digestive tract and into your bloodstream. The type of fat you eat is important – some fats are good for you, while others are best avoided.

Which fats are healthy?

There are two main categories: monounsaturated and polyunsaturated.

Monounsaturated fats are found in olives, canola, peanut oils, avocados and most nuts. They can reduce the risk of cardiovascular disease by lowering blood cholesterol levels (LDL). They are more resistant to oxidation, a process that leads to cell and tissue damage.

Polyunsaturated fats – also known as omega-6 or

omega-3 oils – contain essential fatty acids. Omega-6 is found in corn, sunflower oil and cottonseed oil, while omega-3 is abundant in oily fish – salmon, tuna, trout, mackerel, sardines and herring – and is also present in canola oil, flaxseed and walnuts. Omega-3 relaxes narrowed arteries, reduces the risk of arterial blockages and decreases VLDLs (very low-density lipoproteins – fats in the bloodstream associated with cardio-vascular disease). They may also ease rheumatoid arthritis pain, fight depression and reduce the risk of premature birth.

Which fats should I avoid?

Saturated fat and trans fat. Both have been linked to high cholesterol and heart disease. Saturated fat is found in red meat, dark-meat poultry (with skin) and full-fat dairy products. Trans fat is created when vegetable oil undergoes hydrogenation, a chemical process that extends its shelf life. It is common in fast foods, packaged and convenience foods, snack items (like chips and crackers), cake mixes, pastries, biscuits, shortenings and some margarine.

Limit your intake of both saturated and trans fats by checking the nutrition panel on food labels (trans fats are not always listed but the phrase 'partially hydrogenated oil' is a giveaway – see page 27 for more on food labels).

Try to swap bad fats for good fats – eat salmon instead of steaks and burgers, and pass up the fried food at the lunch bar in favour of tuna or grilled chicken sandwiches. Dip the bread in a little olive oil instead of slathering it with butter or margarine.

Five big fat food fibs

Misconceptions about food have been around forever. Backed by so-called 'experts', some claims sound plausible but rarely have any basis in truth. Here are five common food fibs – and the facts.

Fib: You can eat as much low-fat food as you want without gaining weight.
Fact: Kilojoule for kilojoule, low-fat and full-fat foods are often the same. Food manufacturers often replace the fat in low-fat products with high-kilojoule fruit purees and sugar to make up for the missing flavour. My advice: pay attention to the food's overall energy content, not just the fat.

Fib: Chicken and fish are always low in fat.
Fact: Chicken thighs and legs can be higher in fat than some lean cuts of beef. Eat the skin,

and a chicken dinner becomes a high-fat feast. Cut the fat by choosing white meat – roasted, grilled or steamed – and remove the skin before cooking. Some fish, like mackerel and salmon, are high in fat. This is in the form of valuable omega-3 fatty acids, so do not stint yourself. Cut fat by grilling rather than frying fish.

Fib: Beef is bad for you.
Fact: Beef's reputation has deteriorated because some cuts are high in saturated fat. Lean cuts, however, provide as few as 4 grams of fat per 100-gram trimmed serving. Beef is an excellent source of iron, which is an important protection against anaemia.

Fib: Late-night snacks go straight to your hips and thighs.
Fact: It is true that fewer kilojoules are burned while you

sleep (no matter how much you toss and turn!). It is best to eat your main meal during the day, not at night. Whatever time you eat, if you consume too many kilojoules overall, you will gain weight – on your thighs and everywhere else.

Fib: Carbohydrates make you fat.

Fact: Excess kilojoules are the problem, whether you get them from protein or carbohydrates. Carbohydrates are the body's fuel of choice (at least 50 per cent of your daily intake of kilojoules should be in the form of complex carbs); omitting them is like driving your car without filling the petrol tank.

EATING FOR ENERGY

Food means energy, and Australians are not exactly starving. Why are so many people dragging through the day and crashing by mid-afternoon? Their diets do not provide enough carbohydrates, the body's preferred source of energy. When you eat an apple or a bagel, you effortlessly break down the carbohydrates into glucose (sugar), the body's basic currency unit of energy. Your brain and muscles cannot function without a steady, sustained supply of glucose.

Research has shown that the low-carb, high-fat diets that are currently popular often leave people feeling dull and lethargic, because fat is slow to digest. There are other problems with such diets: they allow virtually unlimited amounts of red meat, bacon, eggs and other fatty foods but limit carbohydrates such as bread, potatoes, most fruits and many vegetables – important sources of cancer-preventing antioxidants and fibre. (See pages 139–46 for my lowdown on popular diets.)

If your energy is flagging, it is time for a well-balanced diet that incorporates the optimum mix of carbohydrates, fats and proteins. Carbohydrates provide a good lift, while fat and protein are digested more slowly, so you get a continuous release of glucose if you spread your intake through several small meals over the course of the day.

Labels

By law, a nutrition panel is required on the packaging of any food product making a nutritional claim (such as that it is low in fat or salt). Some food manufacturers choose to put nutrition panels on their products regardless of whether they are making any such claims. The information on a nutrition panel relates to a standard serve, in addition to a 100-gram serve. Here is an example of what a nutrition panel looks like, and how to interpret it.

Recommended serve size: 30 g		
Servings per package: 33		
	per serve 30 g	per 100 g
Energy	460 kJ	1540 kJ
Protein	3.6 g	12.0 g
Fat	2.8 g	9.2 g
Carbohydrate	20.2 g	67.5 g
Dietary fibre	3.0 g	10.0 g
Cholesterol	Nil	Nil
Sodium	1.2 mg	4.0 mg
Potassium	106 mg	350 mg

Energy	Energy means kilojoules (some labels give both kilojoule and calorie values. 1 calorie = 4.2 kilojoules).
Fibre	3 grams or more per serve is indicative of a good source of fibre.
Fat	Less than 3 grams of fat per 100 grams of food indicates a low-fat product. (You should be aware that fat is also called vegetable oil or fat, animal oil or fat, shortening, copha, lard or tallow, coconut or palm oil and milk solids. Words like 'creamed' or 'toasted' often indicate added fat.)
Sodium	Salt. Less than 120 milligrams per 100 grams indicates a low-salt product. (Salt is also represented as Na+, and is present in Monosodium Glutamate (MSG), sodium bicarbonate, baking powder, baking soda, rock salt and vegetable salt.)
Potassium	A mineral needed to control the working of the muscles and nerves. Ideally, a food product should contain at least as much potassium as sodium.

Other words you might see on nutrition panels or food packages include the following.

Sugar	Can go under a number of names – sucrose, glucose, fructose, maltose, malt extract, honey or molasses.
Cholesterol-free	Plant products do not contain cholesterol. The term 'cholesterol-free' can be misleading, because the food in question could still be high in saturated fat if it contains palm oil or coconut oil. Cholesterol-free does not mean fat-free, as plant fats present in nuts, seeds, avocados and olives will still impact your weight if consumed in excess quantities.

Natural	A general term meaning anything from no pesticides to ice-cream made with milk fat. It does not necessarily equate to 'healthy'.
Light/lite	Used as a marketing tool. It may indicate that the product has less fat, fewer kilojoules, is lower in salt (chips), milder in flavour (olive oil), paler in colour or lighter in texture than related products.
Low-fat/fat reduced	The meaning varies depending on the product. The best way to judge is to compare brands. Remember, 'fat reduced' does not necessarily mean low in fat.
No added salt/ low sodium	The food does not contain added sodium/salt. It might contain natural sodium but the maximum level allowed is 120 milligrams of sodium per 100 grams of the food.

FOUR O'CLOCK LOW

When you are fatigued mid afternoon, avoid the temptation to grab a can of Coke, a glass of orange juice, a cinnamon roll or a big slice of cake in the hope of a quick energy hit. These are carbohydrates, but they will cause your blood sugar level to rise too high and fall too quickly, leaving you right where you started. Ensure you do not overeat when you are tired or stressed. Sit down and eat a healthy snack of protein and carbohydrate – tuna on wholegrain toast, yoghurt with a banana or cheese on a cracker.

Remember: you want to keep your blood sugar level even. When you consume a large portion of carbohydrates –

particularly simple ones – your system responds by secreting a large dose of insulin, the hormone produced in the pancreas. Insulin is responsible for the transport of glucose from the bloodstream into the muscle cells to fuel activity. Provided your pancreas produces the correct amount of insulin when needed, you will feel fine. Unfortunately, many Australians suffer from insulin resistance, meaning that the insulin does not respond exactly as it should. The body compensates for a meal high in simple carbohydrates by secreting more insulin. This causes your blood sugar level to fall, setting off alarms throughout your body.

The main warning bell is adrenaline, the hormone that surges through your veins whenever you sense danger. In this case the peril is not real; your body will prop up blood glucose levels before they fall too far. But the combination of the dip in blood sugar and the jolt of adrenaline can make you feel weak and trembly. You can avoid the jitters by having a high-fibre carbohydrate snack with a moderate amount of protein.

To maintain a high-energy lifestyle: eat small, eat often and choose from a wide variety of foods every day. My eating plan provides three meals and three snacks each day, and is designed to help you feel alert throughout the day.

Weight loss proves a battle of the sexes

Sorry ladies, shedding excess kilos is harder for women than for men. You know the equation: energy in (kilojoules) − energy out (activity and metabolism) = weight lost or gained. For females, this formula is affected by numerous factors; once you understand them, you will comprehend the slower weight loss and accept the action you must take to maintain a healthy weight.

Size matters

In general, women are smaller than men. Consequently, they burn less energy because they do not expend as many kilojoules through metabolism and activity. The larger the person, the more kilojoules they burn because they are moving a greater mass through space.

The hormone effect

Women need a minimum of 12 per cent body fat for their reproductive organs to function efficiently; men need just 4 per cent. Men have more testosterone, a hormone that promotes the development of muscle. Since muscle burns 145–210 kilojoules per 500 grams per day, while fat burns significantly less, a man's more muscular body burns more kilojoules than a woman's, both at rest and during exercise.

Menstruation

The hormonal swings of the menstrual cycle can cause women to yearn for foods high in sugar, fat or salt. Linked to those cravings are emotional highs and lows that can prompt overeating. The more aware you are of the changes that occur during your period, the better equipped you are to develop strategies to deal with them. You might exercise, or schedule a day out of the house to prevent you being tempted to overeat.

Pregnancy

Major hormonal changes can lead to depression, sleep deprivation and overeating, which explains why most women, after delivery, need to lose between 5 and 25 kilograms. Breast-feeding can assist weight loss, because milk production requires 2100 extra kilojoules per day. Many new mums are fatigued and moody, and often give in to overindulgence. However, if they make an effort, they *can* shift the excess kilos gained during pregnancy.

Menopause

At midlife the rate at which women lose lean muscle tissue accelerates. The average adult loses 0.25–0.35 kilograms per year, but as women approach menopause their muscle depletion accelerates to nearly double that rate. This results in their body composition becoming higher in fat and lower in muscle, which significantly reduces their kilojoule-burning potential. In addition, the hormonal changes of menopause causes body fat to be deposited in the abdominal area, resulting in a more male pattern of weight gain. This is *not* inevitable. Research shows that strength and resistance training significantly reduces abdominal fat in older women, while increasing lean muscle tissue.

Reduced intake of kilojoules and regular exercise are other key components to regaining control over your weight and shape, despite your age or stage of life.

CHAPTER 3

Your eating plan

You now know what is required for successful long-term weight loss: consuming fewer kilojoules than you burn. Sounds simple, but the difficult component is developing a pattern of eating you can live with and which will maintain your lighter weight once you have lost the excess kilos. It is important that you realise this will involve changing your lifestyle – both your eating and exercise habits. The majority of people who manage to maintain their weight loss do not follow extreme diets, they increase their physical activity while reducing their intake of fat and kilojoules – and they make this change for the rest of their lives.

The reason many so-called diets fail is because they put certain foods – and often entire food groups – off-limits. A diet that is too restrictive does not set good eating patterns that will last forever. No foods should be avoided completely provided you watch the size of your portions (more on this in Chapter 7), especially those items high in fat and kilojoules. For these ones: go easy, don't go without entirely.

The eating plan included in this chapter will provide all the nutrients required to keep you healthy. There is no such thing as a 'good' or 'bad' food; all foods are broken down within the body and are then used for growth, repair and day-to-day activity. The issue is not any particular type of food – what matters is the quantities you eat and how you balance them in your total intake.

The eating plan provides three meals and three between-meal snacks – morning tea, afternoon tea and supper – to ensure that your energy and blood sugar levels are maintained, as well as a good metabolic rate. All the food groups are included according to the Healthy Food Pyramid (see page 17). You should allow at least an hour between meals and snacks; and you should never go more than three hours without eating.

DON'T COUNT KILOJOULES

While you do have to reduce your overall kilojoule intake to lose weight, kilojoule-counting can become an obsession. It is also quite abstract and removed from the reality of your daily eating, because you are focusing on numbers, not on achieving a healthy nutritional balance. Kilojoule-counting is hard to live with, which is why I want you to start thinking in terms of carbohydrates, proteins and fats – the three food groups that supply the body with the energy, minerals, vitamins and nutrients needed for growth and repair of body tissues. (You will find a list of proteins and carbohydrates on pages 40–43.)

Professional advice

Nutrition needs vary according to individual metabolic rates and other factors, such as activity levels and health status. (For example, a person with diabetes requires an eating plan specific to this health issue.) If you have a health problem or need constant encouragement, I recommend you consult a professional dietician to personalise a program for your individual needs. Typically, at such a consultation, the dietician will weigh and measure you, and will ask about your medical history, eating and exercise habits, lifestyle patterns and history of weight. They will then devise an individual eating and exercise plan and will organise future consultations to track your progress and make adaptations to your present meal plan when necessary.

When you become accustomed to eating according to a meal plan, you will see that it is a simple way to work out your daily intake of proteins, carbohydrates and fats. Instead of endless writing down numbers, you just have to think: 1 protein, 2 carbohydrates (depending on how old you are, your activity level and whether you are male or female – see 'Eating right for your age and gender' on the following page). Do not stress if you find it hard to grasp initially. It is explained in detail in this chapter, and you can see how it works in food terms in the menu planner at the end of the book.

What exactly is a 'serve'? I have outlined this on pages 40–43 with a list of the quantities of various foods that equate to a serve of protein or a serve of carbohydrate. You will also notice a listing of 'free foods'; these are foods high in nutrients, such as vitamins, minerals, fibre and water, and low in kilojoules and fat, such as salad greens and many vegetables. You can enjoy these foods until you feel comfortable; never full and bloated. You must utilise condiments when preparing food, because you want your meals to be tasty and delicious. Low-joule drinks can be consumed liberally – although fresh water is preferable.

EATING RIGHT FOR YOUR AGE AND GENDER

The quantity of carbohydrates and proteins you should eat on a daily basis will depend on a variety of factors, including your age and gender. While individual needs vary, here is a general breakdown of the requirements of teenagers and adults.

Note: Daily allowance for all age groups: 2 cups low-fat milk; 2 teaspoons fat.

Teenage girls (aged 13–19)

Breakfast:	1 protein and 1 carbohydrate; or 2 carbohydrates
Morning tea:	1 carbohydrate
Lunch:	1 protein and 2 carbohydrates
Afternoon tea:	1 carbohydrate
Dinner:	1 protein and 2 carbohydrates
Supper:	1 carbohydrate

or

Breakfast:	1 protein and 1 carbohydrate; o
Morning tea:	1 carbohydrate
Lunch:	1 protein and 2 carbohydrates
Afternoon tea:	1 carbohydrate and 1 protein
Dinner:	1 protein and 1 carbohydrate
Supper:	1 carbohydrate

Teenage boys (aged 13–19)

Breakfast:	1 protein and 2 carbohydrates
Morning tea:	1 carbohydrate
Lunch:	1 protein and 3 carbohydrates
Afternoon tea:	1 protein and 1 carbohydrate
Dinner:	2 proteins and 2 carbohydrates (if they like protein); or 1 protein and 3 carbohydrates
Supper:	1 carbohydrate

Adult women (aged 20–49)

Breakfast:	1 protein and 1 carbohydrate; or 2 carbohydrates
Morning tea:	1 carbohydrate
Lunch:	1 protein and 2 carbohydrates
Afternoon tea:	1 carbohydrate
Dinner:	1 protein and 1 carbohydrate
Supper:	1 carbohydrate

or

Breakfast:	1 protein and 1 carbohydrate; or 2 carbohydrates
Morning tea:	1 carbohydrate
Lunch:	1 protein and 2 carbohydrates
Afternoon tea:	1 carbohydrate and 1 protein
Dinner:	1 protein
Supper:	1 carbohydrate

ult men (aged 20–49)

Breakfast:	1 protein and 1 carbohydrate; or 2 carbohydrates
Morning tea:	1 carbohydrate
Lunch:	1 protein and 3 carbohydrates
Afternoon tea:	1 carbohydrate
Dinner:	2 proteins and 2 carbohydrates; or 1 protein and 3 carbohydrates
Supper:	1 carbohydrate

or

Breakfast:	1 protein and 1 carbohydrate; or 2 carbohydrates
Morning tea:	1 carbohydrate
Lunch:	1 protein and 2 carbohydrates
Afternoon tea:	1 carbohydrate and 1 protein
Dinner:	2 proteins and 2 carbohydrates; or 1 protein and 3 carbohydrates
Supper:	1 carbohydrate

Women aged 50+

Breakfast:	1 carbohydrate
Morning tea:	1 carbohydrate
Lunch:	1 protein and 2 carbohydrates
Afternoon tea:	1 carbohydrate
Dinner:	1 protein and 2 carbohydrates (depending on the level of physical activity; if very inactive, reduce this to 1 protein and 1 carbohydrate)
Supper:	1 carbohydrate

or

Breakfast:	1 carbohydrate
Morning tea:	1 carbohydrate
Lunch:	1 protein and 2 carbohydrates
Afternoon tea:	1 carbohydrate and 1 protein

Dinner:	1 protein and 1 carbohydrate (depending on the level of physical activity; if very inactive, reduce this to 1 protein and 0 carbohydrate)
Supper:	1 carbohydrate

Men aged 50+

Breakfast:	1 protein and 1 carbohydrate; or 2 carbohydrates
Morning tea:	1 carbohydrate
Lunch:	1 protein and 3 carbohydrates
Afternoon tea:	1 carbohydrate
Dinner:	1 protein and 2 carbohydrates; or 2 proteins and 1 carbohydrate
Supper:	1 carbohydrate

Milk, fat and alcohol

As well as thinking in terms of carbohydrate and protein serves, you should consider your daily intake of milk, fat and alcohol. The quantities below apply regardless of age or gender.

Milk

You must have 2 cups of low-fat milk a day to meet your body's requirement of calcium, which keeps bones strong and can help prevent osteoporosis.

Fat

You should restrict your intake of added fat (that is, on top of the fat already present in dairy, meat, chicken, fish and nuts) to 2 teaspoons per day of butter, margarine, cream, oil, peanut butter, avocado, coconut cream, mayonnaise or sour cream.

Alcohol

I recommend you limit your intake of alcohol as much as possible. However, if you enjoy a drink, limit your intake to no more than two standard drinks a day. Keep in mind that 1 standard drink = 1 carbohydrate serve, and may be traded for other carbohydrates.

How much is one serve?

To help you translate one serve of carbohydrate or one serve of protein into real food terms, here is a list of foods that equate to one serve. You will see later how easily you can mix these up to create a meal plan for yourself full of interesting, enticing meals.

1 carbohydrate serve

Fruit

1 apple/5 pieces dried

3 fresh apricots/5 dried halves

1 small banana

1 cup berries

½ cup unsweetened canned fruit

20 cherries

½ small custard apple

3 dates

3 figs/2 dried

½ cup unsweetened fruit juice

½ cup fruit salad

1 grapefruit

15 grapes

1 cup honeydew melon

2 kiwifruit

7 lychees

1 mandarin

1 small mango

1 nectarine

1 medium orange

1 small papaya

5 medium passionfruit

1 large peach

1 pear

2 persimmons

½ cup pineapple

2 medium plums

3 prunes

1 cup rhubarb

1 cup rockmelon

2 tablespoons sultanas/raisins

1 medium tangelo

1 cup cubed watermelon

Vegetables

½ cup baked beans

½ cup corn

1 small corn cob

½ cup creamed corn

½ cup mashed potato

½ cup peas

1 medium potato

1 cup pumpkin

½ cup sweet potato

1 cup thick vegetable soup

Breads and cereals

½ small bagel (30 g)

1 slice bread (30 g)

4 breadsticks (20 g)

⅔ cup buttermilk

⅔ cup cereal

4 corn thins

⅓ cup cooked couscous

½ plain croissant

½ crumpet

plain focaccia (30 g)

2 Ginger Nut Biscuits

2 Marie Biscuits

½ piece matzo

2 Morning Coffee Biscuits

1 cup low-fat milk

2 Milk Arrowroot Biscuits

½ English muffin

⅓ cup cooked pasta/noodles

½ small pita bread

2 cups cooked plain popcorn

½ cup cooked porridge

15 pretzels

1 slice raisin bread

⅓ cup cooked rice

2 thick rice cakes

½ roll (30 g)

2 Shredded Wheatmeal

30 g Turkish bread

10 rice crackers

1 taco shell

1 tortilla (15-centimetre diameter)

1 carton low-fat yoghurt (200 g)

2 Saos/3 Jatz

3 Vitawheat/Crackerbread

4 Water Crackers

Snacks that can be used occasionally as a carbohydrate serve

1 breakfast bar	2 wafers Kit Kat
potato chips (20 g)	1 Le Snack (Uncle Toby's)
3 small squares chocolate (30 g)	3 Liquorice Allsorts
1 scoop plain ice-cream	3 Minties
8 Fruit Pastilles	2 scoops sorbet
1 icy pole	1 Scotch Finger Biscuit
6 jelly babies	1 Tim Tam
6 jelly beans	1 small piece Violet Crumble

1 protein serve

Dairy

5 tablespoons cottage cheese

2.5 cm cube cheese

30 g sandwich slice cheese

3 tablespoons ricotta cheese

30 g fetta cheese

100 g Fruche Lite

1 cup low-fat milk

200 g low-fat yoghurt

Meat

1 rasher lean bacon

1 small chop (lamb/beef/pork)

1 slice ham/roast lamb/beef

½ cup lean mince

1 thin grilled sausage

1 small slice fillet steak (100 g)

1 small slice veal

Seafood

1 medium fillet fish (palm-size)

100 g lobster

12 oysters natural

100 g tin crab

½ cup shelled prawns

100 g sardines, drained

2 thin slices smoked salmon

100 g tin salmon/tuna (in brine
   or spring water)

6 scallops

Poultry

chicken (skin removed):
   ½ breast, 1 leg or 1 thigh

1 small slice turkey

Beans

⅓ cup baked beans

100 g fresh bean curd/tofu

2 tablespoons hummus

½ cup cooked lentils or soya/
  chick/lima beans

Nuts

⅓ cup almonds/walnuts

½ cup cashews/peanuts

1 level tablespoon peanut butter

2 tablespoons tahini

1 egg

3 egg whites

Free foods

(These are foods that you can consume in large but not unlimited quantities – remember, eat only until you are comfortable; never full or bloated.)

Vegetables

alfalfa sprouts

artichokes

asparagus

bean sprouts

beetroot

broccoli

brussels sprouts

cabbage

capers

capsicum

carrot

cauliflower

celeriac

celery

chicory

Chinese greens

choko

cucumber

eggplant

endive

garlic

gherkins

ginger

green beans

leek

lemon

lettuce

marrow

mushroom

onion

parsley

parsnip

peppers

pickled vegetables

radish

sauerkraut

shallots

silver beet

snow peas

spinach
sprouts
squash
tomato
turnip
watercress
zucchini

Drinks

Bonox/beef tea
coffee
low-joule cordials
diet drinks
tea/herbal teas
soda water
stock cubes or Real Stock
tomato juice (1 cup a day)
water/mineral water

Condiments

artificial sweeteners
balsamic vinegar
barbecue sauce
black bean sauce
bran, unprocessed
non-stick cooking spray

curry paste (not satay)
curry powder
fish paste
gelatine
low-joule flavouring (in
    moderation)
herbs and spices
horseradish
lemon
lemon juice
low-joule jelly
mustard
oyster sauce
pepper
relish
no-oil salad dressing
soy sauce
sweet chilli sauce
tomato sauce
teriyaki
vanilla
Vegemite/Promite
vinegar
Worcestershire sauce
yeast

Foods to consume in moderation

(For example a scrape of jam or a drizzle of honey)

Foods rich in sugar or fat – these are concentrated kilojoules and
otherwise low in nutritional value.

Sugar, glucose, honey, marmalade, jam, chutney, syrups, sweet spreads, sweets, chocolates, sweetened canned fruit, jellies, ice-cream, soft drinks, milkshakes, sweetened flavourings for milk, cakes, biscuits and pastries.

Fatty meats, potato chips, mayonnaise, dripping, vegetables baked in fat or fried, fatty soups, gravies and sauces.

HOW TO PUT YOUR EATING PLAN INTO PRACTICE

Soon you will be setting up your own eating plan. To illustrate how this works in practical terms, consider this example for a teenage boy or man. Each day he is allowed:

Breakfast:	1 protein and 2 carbohydrates
Morning tea:	1 carbohydrate
Lunch:	1 protein and 3 carbohydrates
Afternoon tea:	1 protein and 1 carbohydrate
Dinner:	2 proteins and 2 carbohydrates; or 1 protein and 3 carbohydrates
Supper:	1 carbohydrate

So, an example of some options for his daily eating plan is:

For breakfast:
- 1 poached egg (1 protein) on 2 slices of toast (2 carbohydrates), with grilled mushrooms (free) and tomato (free), or
- 100 g baked beans (1 protein) on 2 slices of toast (2 carbohydrates).

For lunch:
- 1 sandwich (2 slices bread = 2 carbohydrates) with 120 g chicken breast (1 protein) and salad (free), seasoned with mustard or pickles, and 1 piece of fruit (1 carbohydrate), or

- 2 cups thick vegetable soup (2 carbohydrates), seasoned with mixed herbs, black pepper or Tabasco, 1 slice of bread (1 carbohydrate) and a 200 g low-fat yoghurt (1 protein), or
- 200 g baked potato (2 carbohydrates) with cottage cheese (1 protein) and salad (free), plus 1 piece of fruit (1 carbohydrate).

For dinner:
- 1 palm-sized serve of grilled fish (1 protein) prepared with sweet chilli sauce, ⅔ cup cooked rice (2 carbohydrates) and green salad (free) with stir-fried vegetables, plus 1 scoop of ice-cream (1 carbohydrate) or
- 2 lamb chops (2 proteins), 1 jacket potato (1 carbohydrate), 1 cup cooked pumpkin (1 carbohydrate) and steamed vegetables (free).

Between-meal snacks might be a single carbohydrate. He could choose from:
- 1 piece of fruit
- 200 g low-fat yoghurt
- 1 slice of toast with a smear of jam/honey/Vegemite
- 2 rice cakes with tomato (free) and cracked pepper (free).

These are just a few examples. There are hundreds of possible variations for the combinations of protein and carbohydrate serves, which makes the eating plan flexible to any situation, whether you are at home, at work, out for a meal or dining at a friend's place.

YOUR DAILY EATING PLAN
Now that you know how to structure an interesting, balanced eating plan, I would like you to put together your own plan, depending into which of the age/gender categories you fall.

First, work out your daily allowance of carbohydrates and proteins, and mark them on the table below.

My daily allowance of protein and carbohydrates

Breakfast	_____	serves of protein
	_____	serves of carbohydrate
Morning tea	_____	serves of carbohydrate
Lunch	_____	serves of protein
	_____	serves of carbohydrate
Afternoon tea	_____	serves of protein
	_____	serves of carbohydrate
Dinner	_____	serves of protein
	_____	serves of carbohydrate
Supper	_____	serves of carbohydrate

My daily allowance of milk, fat and alcohol

Fat	_____	teaspoons butter/margarine/cream/oil/ peanut butter/avocado/coconut cream/ mayonnaise/sour cream
Milk	_____	cups Skim/Shape/Lite White/Farmer's Best/Regular/Soy Milk Lite/Dairy Farmers Life Low-Fat
Alcohol	_____	serves per day

Now that you have worked out your allowances, why not put together a few sample menus, based on the carbohydrate and protein serves you have just read through?

TRADING PLACES

The joy of this eating plan is that you can eat what you feel like, as long as you remain within the framework of the portions allowed. For example, if you are a woman and you want to go out for lunch, you know you can have 1 protein and 2 carbohydrates. If you went to a seafood restaurant, your allowance could equate to a piece of grilled fish, a jacket potato, salad and a slice of bread. However, if you felt like having dessert with lunch, you could trade the slice of bread for a small fruit salad, a scoop of ice-cream or a small friand with your coffee. Alternatively, you might choose to trade the potato for a glass of wine. The flexibility is endless.

Examine the list of proteins and carbohydrates on pages 40–43; each item equates to a single serve, and you can mix and match within each category (that is, you can only exchange carbohydrate serves for other carbohydrate serves, and protein serves for other protein serves).

Once you are familiar with this system, it becomes very easy and user-friendly. You can work it out when you are planning a meal just by thinking in terms of carbohydrates or proteins that are permitted at that particular meal.

RING UP THE CHANGES

You can vary this eating plan according to your preferences or lifestyle, as long as you stay within your daily allowance of carbohydrates and proteins. If you prefer more carbohydrate at breakfast, you could opt for 2 carbohydrates then, instead of 1 carbohydrate and 1 protein.

Many women and teenage girls do not like a big dinner; others experience a mid-afternoon slump in energy. They could opt for a substantial mid-afternoon snack, adding a protein serve to their afternoon tea (for example, a slice of cheese or 100 g tin of tuna on toast served with a salad), and subtracting a carbohydrate serve from their dinner.

If you like to go to bed early, you could skip supper and have an extra carbohydrate for dinner instead.

You can also indulge yourself with the occasional treat within the framework of this eating plan. For example, you might be yearning for something sweet; you could exchange one of your carbohydrate serves (not more than once a day) for three liquorice allsorts, a scoop of plain ice-cream or three small squares of chocolate. You cannot make the exchange for a 'treat' more than once a day, because such treats are lower in nutrients and fibre than bread, fruit, vegetables or other carbohydrates.

You can also swap a carbohydrate serve for a standard alcoholic drink. For example, you might exclude a carbohydrate serve with dinner for a glass of white wine. Watch your alcohol intake and never exceed more than two drinks in one day – so if you do not drink for several days, this does not mean you can save up and binge drink!

HUNGER IS YOUR FRIEND

You will find the eating plan difficult for the first four weeks. You have to continually refer to the tables to determine the different food types, but eventually it becomes part of your memory bank. In addition, you might feel hungry for the first four weeks, because your body is used to snacking and eating larger meals, so it has to adapt. When your appetite, hunger signals and metabolism get back into sync, you will feel hungry at meal times — which is expected and normal.

Hunger is a common feeling; it is your body's cue to eat. However, it is one with which many people are unfamiliar because they have been overeating for so long. Frequently their hunger cues are out of sync because they are used to eating to a schedule, not appetite. Often they are not hungry in the morning — when they should be — and skip breakfast. They will be very hungry at dinner, simply because they are used to eating a big meal at this time.

It will take about a month before your appetite normalises. Then when you wake up in the morning you should feel hungry and be ready for breakfast. In fact, you should feel hungry for every meal. If, once your appetite has normalised, you do not feel hungry before a meal, this suggests that you may have eaten more than your requirement at the previous meal. You have probably increased your portion sizes and you need to reduce your daily intake. Never omit breakfast or meals early in the day, rather leave out the carbohydrates at dinner.

Many people are terrified of feeling hungry. But remember, as long as you stick to a healthy eating plan, hunger is a natural instinct. It tells you when to eat and when to stop eating. You need to get in touch with your appetite — to be hungry at every meal, and eat only until you are satisfied, not bloated.

On a brighter note, people often tell me that they are not as hungry as they expected on this eating plan, because they are eating every three hours, so their hunger doesn't build to intolerable levels – and you know that your next meal is not such a long wait away!

TAKE IT SLOWLY

Aim for a regular weight loss of 2–2½ kilograms each month – this allows your body to adjust to your new eating and exercise habits without slowing down your metabolic rate, as crash diets can do. Some weeks you will lose more than you do in others, but overall your weight loss should average out at approximately ½ kilogram per week. This means it could take time to reach a weight you are comfortable with. Be patient – you will get to your desired weight with time, but you are learning correct eating and exercise habits, which you will practise forever. Recognise when you have reached a realistic weight for your height and bone structure.

Move it to lose it

The eating plan alone is not sufficient for healthy weight loss. You also have to exercise for at least 45 minutes each day. Aim to walk a minimum of 10 000 steps every day; a pedometer is a terrific motivator and assists you keeping track of your activity level. You can also try yoga, Pilates or weights – but this is in addition to the 10 000 steps you clock up every day. This applies whether you are male or female, young or old – unless, of course, you find movement difficult due to arthritis or other medical problem. (In these cases you might be able to swim or do aqua-aerobics.) The vital role played by exercise is discussed in more detail in Chapter 13.

CHAPTER **4**

Getting started

This is the moment of truth. You now have to commence making permanent lifestyle changes. Altering entrenched habits takes time, perseverance and commitment, and it can be uncomfortable and disorienting. How do you get motivated to eat a healthy diet and exercise regularly – and how do you ensure that you'll maintain these adjustments?

The toughest mindset change is from 'diet' to 'lifestyle'. You must work at this continually; it will take time before the change starts to pay dividends.

It's easy for your motivation to falter when you are not seeing obvious results. How to overcome these negative feelings? Acknowledge them. Once you tell yourself it is normal to feel anxious or temporarily discouraged about your efforts to lose weight, you are liberated from the pressure of expecting instant success. You won't beat yourself up for craving chips rather than carrots, or feeling unenthusiastic about exercise, and you won't give yourself a hard time over the occasional splurge.

> *'A journey of a thousand miles must begin with a single step'*
>
> ━
>
> CHINESE PROVERB

Being overweight is a state of mind, and the body reflects this loss of psychological and physical balance; it does take time to restore that balance. Be aware that change is unsettling, and expect to take it slowly – week by week. As your eating becomes more controlled, you will feel stronger, more energetic and confident – and you will achieve a better balance in your life.

MAKE A RESOLUTION

It is not enough to want to lose weight, you have to have an action plan or it's not going to happen. Start by making a pact with yourself, and write it down. Tell someone you trust about your goal, because public disclosure can be a more powerful motivator than private commitment – it makes you accountable to somebody other than yourself. Choose someone supportive who you know will encourage you and not give you a hard time when things aren't going to plan. Conversely, you might feel this is a private problem you would like to overcome alone.

CONSIDER THE HEALTH BENEFITS

The immediate pleasure experienced in losing weight is simply looking and feeling better – your reflection in the mirror emphasises that all the hard work has been worth it! It is

'Seeing' your success

Visualisation is a useful psychological tool that can help you attain your goals. It involves seeing yourself in your mind's eye as you would like to be – slimmer, more organised, competent in your chosen sphere, or whatever your particular objective might be. Make your vision as real as possible, imagining how you will feel and look when you are where you want to be. File this mental snapshot in your memory and revisit it regularly as the months go by and you grow closer to your weight-loss objectives. It will help inspire you and keep you on track.

wonderful to be able to shop for clothes you like, as opposed to clothes you buy to disguise your figure.

There is, however, an additional incentive that should keep you on track whenever you feel your motivation flagging: the dramatic health benefits of shedding the excess weight. Dropping kilos reduces the risk of developing several serious illnesses over the long term. Here are some examples to show you how much more your body will love you when it is at a healthy weight.

Type 2 diabetes
Type 2 diabetes is becoming more prevalent among the overweight, obese and inactive. It typically strikes after the age of 50, but it is increasingly being seen among younger people

due to their sedentary lifestyle. Type 2 (mature-age onset) diabetes results from the inability of the body to efficiently utilise insulin, a hormone secreted by the pancreas to remove glucose (sugar) from the bloodstream and transport it to the body's cells to fuel activity. Excess weight appears to interfere with insulin's ability to be sufficiently effective, resulting in high blood glucose (sugar) levels, which requires medication and possibly insulin injections. Uncontrolled high blood glucose levels can lead to unnecessary complications such as blindness, peripheral neuropathy, kidney problems and heart disease. Losing weight and participating in extra activity (exercise) could help prevent the problem from developing — particularly in people with a family history of type 2 diabetes, which is hereditary.

High blood fats

Cholesterol and triglycerides are lipids (fatty substances) produced by the liver and present in the blood. While they are necessary for normal body function, excess triglycerides and cholesterol can result in the formation of plaque deposits in the arteries, blocking them over time and increasing the risk of heart attack and stroke. There are two types of cholesterol: LDL, the 'bad' cholesterol responsible for the damage; and HDL, the 'good' cholesterol that actually removes the bad cholesterol from the vessels and takes it to the liver to be processed. Exercise and weight affect the production of these blood fats. Exercise and weight loss help the levels of triglycerides and LDL in the body to fall, and HDL to increase – your risk factors for heart disease are therefore reduced with an improved lifestyle.

High blood pressure

Blood pressure is a measurement of how hard the heart must work to pump blood around the body. It tends to rise with age and excess weight (because the heart has to work harder to pump blood around a bigger body mass). High blood pressure is associated with serious health problems, including stroke and heart disease. It is treated with medication and lifestyle changes. Losing weight and exercise help lower blood pressure and could keep you off medication.

Cardiovascular disease

Obesity can lead to strokes and heart disease, because it increases the risk factors – high blood pressure, diabetes and high cholesterol – for these killer diseases. Fat accumulation around the midriff (the so-called 'apple shape' typical of overweight men and post-menopausal women) is particularly dangerous. Increasing waist circumference increases the risks of developing heart disease in both women and men. While women are protected by oestrogen, post-menopausal women no longer have this hormonal protection, so their risk gradually draws level with men.

Cancer

Colon cancer, ovarian cancer, cervical cancer, prostate cancer and kidney cancer have been linked to obesity. It is also implicated in the development of breast cancer, because fat cells secrete oestrogen – fatter women have higher levels of oestrogen in their bloodstream, which increases their risk of developing hormone-driven breast cancer.

Arthritis and joint pain

Excess weight is associated with the development of arthritis. Excess weight puts further wear and tear on your joints, in addition to straining your muscles. Every few kilograms of weight loss relieves the pressure on your joints and improves your ability to move without pain.

Gallstones

Gallstones form in the gall bladder and are most common in women over 40. Gallstones are formed from bile, a liquid secreted by the liver and stored in the gall bladder, which aids digestion. Bile is by and large made up of cholesterol. Excess cholesterol production increases the risk of gallstones, as does obesity. Intense pain can result if gallstones block the ducts leading from the gall bladder or liver. Reduction of fat in the diet and *gradual* weight loss decrease the risk.

TAKE IT EASY

Although it might seem a good idea to dive headfirst into a weight-loss program and lifestyle change, it can be a road to disappointment. Anyone who works out at a gym is familiar with those novices who sign on for an over-ambitious program, full of enthusiasm. The first few weeks they go at

The will to win

Question: I have always been a big girl but now my weight is getting to a point where my health is affected. I am scared I could have a heart attack. I have tried to diet before and it just hasn't worked. Any advice?

Answer: You have to really want to alter your lifestyle to lose weight. Fear can certainly be an incentive, but actions speak louder than words – especially if your weight is impacting your health. I suggest you seek professional advice from a dietician to structure an eating and exercise plan for you, and to monitor your progress. It is essential that you look at long-term changes, not quick fixes. Don't focus on weight loss; rather, make small changes weekly and eventually you will notice the kilos falling off. More importantly, you will have developed better habits. Believe me, you will be successful if you have the right attitude.

it hell-for-leather, but by the fifth or sixth week they have injured themselves or have burned out. They have sabotaged themselves simply by overdoing it. So, how to avoid becoming a weight-loss casualty?

Build on your successes

As the old saying goes, 'Anything you can do a little of, you can do a lot of'. Start by making small changes and then build on them. In weight loss, as with other endeavours, simply getting started is half the battle. As you enjoy the results – and you will, if you maintain smaller portions of low-fat foods and begin an exercise regime – you will be even more committed to building on your achievements! Success breeds more commitment.

Hang in there . . .

There are many reasons why weight-loss regimes backfire, but one often-overlooked pitfall is unrealistic expectations. Here is where some commonsense comes in. Contrary to what some fad diets may claim, no-one loses 5 kilograms in a week. Nor is it likely to have been gained over such a short timeframe. If it took you five years to put on the excess, it's unlikely to disappear in five weeks. There are no quick fixes in weight loss – it's the continuous daily effort that makes the difference. Remember, a lapse is not a failure – tomorrow is another day to be positive and to change those entrenched habits.

Stick to the eating plan I've outlined in the previous chapter. Whatever progress you see on the bathroom scale or from the fit of your clothes – no matter how small – shows that you are on the right track.

And forget the past

If you have a history of trying and failing to lose weight, put it behind you. Learn from your mistakes, and remind yourself that this time you *will* succeed. You *will* make better choices; you *will* keep your portions small; and you *will* exercise regularly. Most importantly, the changes you implement are forever!

Remember that the odd splurge does not spell the end of your efforts (it could even be crucial to ultimate success), and it is normal – you cannot be perfect all the time, no-one is. Don't be too rigid. If you give yourself the leeway to experiment to find what works best for you, you will end up with better, lasting results. Don't give up! Just do your best and you will succeed.

CHAPTER **5**

THE FIRST COMMANDMENT:

A lifestyle, not a diet

Losing weight isn't easy. It requires planning, perseverance and, more importantly, a psychological shift from thinking in terms of short-term diets to long-term changes in total lifestyle. Changing your eating style is one ingredient of the weight-loss equation. It is a commitment involving changing your life in numerous ways, including increasing your physical activity, making time for yourself, enjoying your family and relationships, socialising and bringing a balance of all these facets to your life.

I do not like to use the word 'diet', because it implies short-term deprivation and an unnecessary punishment. I would like you to stop dieting now. Does this seem an odd commandment to commence with? Considering you bought this book because you are looking for the ultimate 'diet', right? Wrong. If you think like this, you are likely to have a struggle shedding the excess kilos, only to have them eventually creep back on again. Attaining and maintaining a healthy weight is not a short-term goal, it requires a lifetime plan.

Forget thinking about 'diet foods'. When you think of the term, do you think of cottage cheese, yoghurt, eggs, lettuce, grapefruit, celery, tuna and carrots? Many people do until they cannot bear the sight of yoghurt or cottage cheese, or whatever the mainstay is of the diet they have been on lately. All food should be varied, nutritious and delicious. I want you to make a commitment to a healthier lifestyle, not to a temporary, quick-fix diet.

Most people who yearn to lose weight believe that all they have to do is eat less or eat differently for a brief period of time until they achieve their goal weight. Once the weight is lost, they revert to their old eating habits. The diet is over and everything is back to normal.

Everything *is* back to normal: they are soon back to their old weight, and usually even heavier. Then they embark on another diet, lose weight, lapse, and the cycle continues. This is classic yo-yo dieting, which is unhealthy and counter-productive both physically and psychologically.

THE PERILS OF YO-YO DIETING

Yo-yo dieting – taking weight off, putting it on again, and then trying to take it off once more – is an endless, emotionally draining battle. After repeated stringent dieting, the body changes, becoming more efficient at hoarding energy and storing it as fat. Lethargy is common. Normal activities – sitting, exercising and even sleeping – use fewer kilojoules. Any future very-low-kilojoule dieting results in slower weight loss despite the body consuming exactly the same number of kilo-joules as during previous regimes. A slower metabolic rate is also a side effect of repeated dieting.

A study discovered that in order for yo-yo dieters to maintain their lighter weight, they could only consume an average intake of 5451 kilojoules a day, whereas people under normal eating and exercise controls could consume 8190 kilojoules a day to stay at their new weight. It's no wonder that a sizeable number of yo-yo dieters not only relapse, but become even heavier than they were previously, because their bodies require less energy to achieve the same results.

The 'thrifty gene syndrome' can be explained biologically, because we have evolved from animals that need to be able to conserve energy and fat to tide them over in lean times. When famine strikes, the body defends its fat reserves by slowing its metabolic rate. We now live in a time of plenty, when it is easy to overeat and grow fat. Then, when we diet to shed the excess, our bodies cannot differentiate between natural famine and the self-inflicted variety (a low-kilojoule diet). The more frequently we repeat the feast–famine cycle, the more efficient our metabolism becomes . . . and the better at storing fat and conserving energy. Consequently, yo-yo dieting is not just ineffective over the long term, it can leave you fatter despite eating less!

GETTING OFF THE DIET CAROUSEL

Yo-yo dieting has not only a detrimental physical effect on you, but also a destructive psychological impact. Continual starting and stopping with different diets will warp your attitude towards food. Far from being an essential and enjoyable part of life, it becomes an object of fear with a disturbing and disproportionate influence over your behaviour. It controls you, rather than you controlling it. Instead of sustaining you, it fills you with guilt, helplessness and other negative feelings. These undesirable emotions encourage out-of-control eating, bingeing and starving; and so the diet carousel keeps turning. It's time to get off!

Dieting doesn't work. Changing your lifestyle does. You must modify your mindset. This can be difficult for many people who have been on one diet or another for so long that they do not know what normal eating is. Consider Josie, 35, an office manager. Over the past twenty years, Josie has been on high-fibre diets, low-carb diets, detox regimes or diets based on various supplements or special foods. In fact, she cannot remember a period during this time when she was not trying to restrict her food intake. Despite spending time and money keeping up with all these diets, Josie often falls short of whatever they demand. She has lost weight and gained weight, but overall nothing much has changed, apart from her attitude to food. She feels that it is something she cannot be trusted with; just thinking about her next meal causes her anxiety. She considers herself a failure – but she still believes that if she could discover the perfect diet 'for her', she would ultimately succeed.

Does this sound like you? You are not alone; it is common, particularly with women. You have to change your attitude if you are going to achieve your goal of losing weight and keeping it off. Flick the switch from negative to positive thinking. In a society obsessed with slimness, it is not easy to change from a diet mentality to one that emphasises a lifestyle of healthy eating and a positive body image. Start by making a commitment to your own wellbeing. You are choosing to improve your health and nutrition, by eating more fruit and vegetables, and less fat. It is something you select to do, not something imposed on you, which is why you are willing to incorporate the necessary changes into your life, and are determined to persevere over the long haul. You will lapse at times; this is normal! Remind yourself that you are not a failure; no-one is successful all the time.

Keep a food diary

Write down everything you eat. This makes you accountable to yourself and it also discourages mindless eating, which can add hundreds of unnoticed kilojoules to your daily intake. Record whatever you have eaten within 15 minutes of doing so, and make sure you carry your diary around with you, so you don't miss a morsel. Do not forget to include snacks, little tastes and nibbles – including finishing off the kids' crusts from lunch and picking while preparing meals. Low-fat or regular milk? Baked or fried chicken? Note when, what and how much you ate, as well as your main reason for eating (such as hunger, boredom or loneliness).

This will help identify patterns relating to emotional eating (see page 76), making it easier to introduce strategies to address them. It will also help you gauge the balance in your life.

Here's an example of a diary to get you started.

Date: _____

Time: _____

What I ate/quantity: _____

How I felt: _____

What exercise I did today:_____

What other satisfying activities I engaged in today:

_____

_____

_____

_____

BELIEVE IN YOURSELF

Permanent weight loss can seem impossible when you hear over and over again how many people lose weight only to eventually regain it. What you don't hear, though, is about the people who have lost weight and kept it off. These people do not just alter the way they eat and exercise, they modify their minds. They believe in themselves, and so must you. To help you keep this in mind, I have included some success stories from some of my clients, written by them to share their experiences and help keep you on track.

> *'It is not the mountains that we conquer, but ourselves'*
>
> —
>
> SIR EDMUND HILLARY

Success requires you to visualise yourself as capable of achieving, maintaining and being comfortable at a healthy weight. Faith in your own abilities and capacities will enable you to achieve your objectives. However, many overweight people lack the confidence that they can ever be slim. They have had so many failures that they expect to fail, and this expectation can become self-fulfilling. You must challenge every expectation and convince yourself you can succeed.

People who believe their weight problems were caused by their own choices – what they choose to eat and how they choose to exercise – rather than genetics are more likely to shed the excess. They see themselves as in control of their own bodies, and can therefore lose weight if they choose to change their lifestyles. I need you to adopt this attitude.

The bottom line: if you think you can lose weight, you will. You are in charge of your eating. You have chosen to buy, cook and eat the food you have been eating until now, so you *can* alter your eating. You might have tried and failed before, but this has no impact on the future. Challenge your assumptions!

STAYING MOTIVATED

How do you stay positive and motivated in the long term? Entrenched habits of eating and lack of exercise are difficult

Larry, 38, engineer

Larry had been overweight since he was a teenager and assumed he would always be fat. He once said, 'When I lose weight'; after a while, he stopped even thinking it, because his obesity was here to stay. Nothing changed for twenty years except that Larry grew heavier. Then he had a health scare. His blood pressure shot up and he discovered that his cholesterol was too high. 'My GP was great,' Larry says. 'She advised me to lose weight but she didn't read me the riot act. She referred me to a dietician, who really encouraged me and convinced me that I could succeed.' Larry has done it. He has dropped 20 kilograms and plans to lose another 10 kilograms – and he is confident he can do it. As he says, 'Having someone supportive behind me made an enormous difference – and the positive reinforcement of my blood pressure dropping, my cholesterol normalising and feeling more energetic, fit and confident motivates me to maintain this new lifestyle.'

to change and require hard work. Understand that when you make changes, you should not expect to feel good immediately. Changing your way of life can be tough, especially since it can take time before your new behaviours start to pay dividends. It can be disheartening to turn up to a party and have to pass on a lot of the goodies on offer. It can be very tempting to give in, particularly if the scales seem to be saying that nothing encouraging is happening. Why miss out on instantaneous gratification for the sake of a future goal – reaching your desired weight – that requires strict adherence to your new eating plan? Sooner or later you are going to lapse. Firstly, you *can* have the food on offer, but keep the portions small – have a taste and leave the rest (more on this topic in Chapter 8). Secondly, and more importantly, don't be rigid; you are setting yourself up for failure. The process of losing weight seems so enormous and overwhelming, the prospect of keeping indefinitely on track seems almost impossible.

Just taking the first positive step – even one as minor as passing up a second helping or going for a walk at lunchtime – will kick-start your motivation. As you see results – and you will, if you follow the advice in this book – you will become increasingly committed to building on your success.

REMAIN OPTIMISTIC

If you believe that staying at your current weight or even gaining more is inevitable, that defeatist attitude increases the likelihood that you won't put in the effort necessary to make changes. If you view yourself as a success, then you will bring more energy into your weight-loss efforts.

CREATE A SELF-FULFILLING PROPHECY

You will stay motivated if you imagine yourself at your goal weight by a nominated time. Having a defined timeline will help focus your efforts. Be realistic. Your self-confidence will increase and you will become more proactive in changing your eating and exercise habits to support your positive self-image.

SET GOALS

Identifying and setting goals is essential to achieving any objective, and losing weight is no exception. Your goals should be as specific as possible – 'I want to lose 10 kilograms', not 'I would like to be slim'. It helps to have short-term goals as well as a long-term objective, because every small success you have along the way boosts your confidence that you can attain your ultimate goal. You must be realistic, or you are setting yourself up for failure. It is not reasonable to plan to

Weigh it up

People who regularly weigh themselves are more likely to keep lost kilos from creeping back. This does not mean you should keep jumping on and off the scales; a weekly weigh-in is sufficient. Weigh yourself on the same scales at the same time of day each week, wearing the same clothing, and record the results. If they are not what you would like, do not judge yourself too harshly; it is just a number, after all, not a moral judgement! If your weight has gone up, it simply means there have been more kilojoules going in than activity going out, and the reason you are reading this book now is to learn how to balance this equation.

lose 10 kilograms in a fortnight, whatever certain magazines might claim; it *is* realistic to aim for a loss of ½ kilogram a week (or 2–2½ kilograms in a month).

Did you ever promise yourself that you would never eat chocolate again? Have you vowed to start running 5 kilometres every day, when you are normally inactive? These are both examples of unrealistic goals that you are unlikely to achieve. Setting yourself these challenges is counterproductive, because all-or-nothing goals encourage all-or-nothing behaviour. You are leaving yourself no room for error or gradual improvement, increasing the risk that you will give up, and consequently increasing your sense of failure. If your downfall is cheesecake, a far more realistic goal – one that you are likely to achieve – would be to limit yourself to one small serving of cheesecake a week rather than denial forever.

Focus on short-term objectives rather than long-term desires. Ask yourself what you can achieve today. It might be cutting out that mid-afternoon chocolate bar, or using the stairs instead of the lift. However inconsequential it may seem, a small achievement every day adds up to big gains over time.

Replace 'I will be' with 'I will do' goals. You might *want to be* slimmer or fitter, but what are you going to *do* to get there? Make your objectives specific – 'I will reduce the size of my food portions', or 'I will walk four times a week'. You have converted a vague wish into a concrete action plan.

Base your current goals on now, not where you hope to be in the future. If you have always eaten a big bowl of ice-cream for dessert, you could assuage your sweet tooth by having fruit for dessert at dinnertime and then a cup of low-fat frozen yoghurt later.

Above all, accept your body type. Humans come in many different shapes and sizes. You should make the most of your inherited characteristics. However, it is unrealistic to aspire to look like Kate Moss or Nicole Kidman, because very few people have their particular genetic make-up (and even fewer have access to the army of beauticians, hairdressers, photographers and fashion designers dedicated to keeping them looking gorgeous; models and film stars often don't look as good in real life as they are made to look in the glossy magazines!). Do not focus on what you cannot change; concentrate on the differences you *can* make.

AND REMEMBER . . .

People who succeed in achieving their weight-loss goals have just as many slip-ups as those who fail. The difference is how you perceive those lapses. Losing weight is a marathon, not a quick sprint. Establishing new attitudes and behaviours takes time and continued practice. You are in this for the long haul, so do not stress if you do not always live up to your new eating plan. If you do have a binge, forgive yourself. Everybody slips occasionally; accept it is quite normal. Forgive yourself and move on. You are not a failure, you are human!

Practise a technique called 'Thought-stopping': the minute a negative thought arises, visualise a stop sign to immediately cut off that thought and then substitute a positive thought to

Recharge and resist

Question: I really want to lose weight but I keep relapsing. How can I boost my willpower?

Answer: Don't feel too bad if you have a second or even a third slice of cake – your resolve is bound to run out at some point. The good news is that it can be replenished. People tend to view willpower as a kind of mental muscle, so failing to use it leaves you feeling like a moral wimp. Do not give yourself a hard time if you overindulge, give yourself a break. The best way to recharge your resolve is to rest. Like every other part of you, your willpower needs time out to revive. Once you are rested and refreshed, you will be better able to deal with temptation.

replace the negative one. For example, if you catch yourself thinking, 'I am hopeless, I simply cannot lose weight', think: 'I am a worthwhile person and I am going to give this my very best shot'. This introduces hope – a powerful antidote to stress. Thought-stopping might sound a little artificial at first, but with regular practice it becomes automatic, and your thinking becomes more optimistic.

SEEK SUPPORT

You do not have to go it alone. Why not enlist support from someone you know will encourage your efforts and keep you going when your motivation flags? This could be your mother, partner, relative or friend. That is a strategy that proved effective for Suzie, 28, a homemaker. She just could not stop herself picking food when the children came home from school. She would make them afternoon tea and then eat what they left

> 'You must do the thing you think you cannot do'
>
> ―
>
> ELEANOR ROOSEVELT

because she did not want to waste it. Often, she would eat what was left in their lunchboxes as well. So Suzie made a pact with her neighbour, Jane, who had a similar problem: instead of heading straight for home after school – and grazing in front of the television with the children – they decided to take the kids to the park instead. They packed snacks for everyone. Suzie and Jane played games with the children. The positive outcome was that they were eating less and moving more than they did at home. The companionship and physical activity was great for everyone!

Sometimes support might not be forthcoming from those closest to you, which is why I recommend seeking professional advice. Dieticians are experts in food and nutrition issues, and are trained to help you identify unhealthy eating patterns and establish better ones. To locate a dietician, contact the Dietitians Association of Australia (www.daa.asn.au).

Overcoming emotional eating

To become chronically overweight, you have been eating for reasons other than genuine hunger. For many people, emotional eating – placating feelings with food – begins in childhood. You hurt your knee, throw a tantrum – a lolly solves everything! So begins the association of food with consolation, rewards or other situations unrelated to nutrition or hunger.

You eat for a variety of reasons – to celebrate a special occasion, to fulfil expectations (such as at a business lunch with a client), out of habit, to alleviate boredom or perhaps to 'medicate' yourself against anxiety, loneliness or depression. Eating may seem easier than attempting to face the underlying psychological issues. Overeating does not help, and usually leaves you feeling awful, guilty and uncomfortable – emotions you should not have to suffer. Bingeing affects your mood, which impacts those around you. Why should innocent children, friends and often a partner experience your changes in temperament due to your bad eating habits? It is often necessary to seek professional assistance when the issues are too complicated to overcome alone. You could start with your GP or dietician, who might refer you to a psychologist or other professional for help.

Identifying and dealing with all the complex and varied issues that cause overeating is a huge topic, outside the scope of this book. As a rule of thumb, to help you clarify your feelings when the urge to eat when you are not hungry strikes, ask yourself these five questions.

1. *What is going on?* Try to identify what is affecting you at that moment.

2. *What do I feel?* Dig deeper to identify your emotional needs and their causes.

3. *What do I need and want?* Figure out what you can do instead of engaging in mindless eating.

4. *What is in my way?* Look at your life to identify any psychological barriers preventing you from changing.

5. *What will I do?* Set goals, keep promises to yourself and maintain your commitment.

Eating patterns are often entrenched habits – something you do whether you are happy, sad, bored, socialising or alone reading or watching television.

Keep a food diary (see page 66) to help you identify your emotional state while eating, and try to think of ways to change conditions that trigger bingeing. Analyse all your relationships and, if you feel that your needs for love, support and affection are not being met, consider ways to express them more effectively. Never eat unless you are relaxed, sitting down and enjoying your food – bingeing and overeating only result in you feeling guilt-ridden, frustrated and disappointed. When you are frazzled remove yourself from the food source – go for a walk, visit a friend, give yourself a manicure, and if you are tired, go to sleep! Fatigue is a major reason for overeating or choosing the wrong types of food.

Explore relaxation techniques – deep breathing,

yoga, visualisation or meditation – to help calm feelings of grief, anxiety, panic, helplessness or hostility (see page 209 for more on these). Keeping a journal can help you understand these feelings; simply expressing them, even if it's only to yourself, on paper, can help the process of dispelling them.

Rising levels of the stress hormone cortisol spur increases in appetite, especially for carbohydrates and fat. So once you have identified how and when you use food to deal with your emotions, determine other ways of addressing feelings of vulnerability, hopelessness and defeat. List the situations, people and activities that make you feel fulfilled, happy, valued or occupied, and make an effort to engage in them regularly. Here is a list of activities you might enjoy.

* Sports: fly a kite, walk, play netball, soccer or tennis
* Art and craft: try ceramics, painting, tapestry or cross-stitch
* Spend time with your family
* Talk to friends
* Devote time to your garden
* Get a pet: pets offer unconditional love and are a constant companion
* Get involved: volunteer for community work, join a choir or sign up for a class
* Pamper yourself: have a facial, manicure or massage, buy yourself flowers
* Take time out for you: visit an art gallery, go to a movie, read a book, do nothing at all!

SUMMING UP . . .

* Think of your eating plan in terms of a healthy lifestyle, not a short-term diet.
* Put your concerns about food, eating and even yourself onto a positive track, increasing your optimism and boosting your motivation.
* Set concrete goals, ensuring they are realistic and sensible, and you are on the path to success.

SUCCESS STORY
Anna

In 1999 I weighed 58 kilograms and was a size 8–10. I moved from Sydney to Melbourne to be with my fiancé, where I suffered a number of setbacks. I left my fiancé when I realised he wasn't the man I thought he was. I then suffered from hormonal problems and glandular fever. I began to gain weight when my doctor placed me on hormone replacement therapy due to a complete lack of oestrogen. I was also eating as a salve to ease my emotional pain and loneliness following my relationship break-up. At work I had to pretend nothing was wrong, and eating helped me to do this. These combined problems sparked off a period of deep depression, which brought up childhood issues and masses of self-loathing. To cope, I was taking antidepressant medication and also started abusing alcohol. My weight escalated further and after three years I weighed 78 kilograms.

I returned to Sydney and began intensive therapy with a psychiatrist. My alcohol abuse was easing. My body was not able to tolerate antidepressants for any extended period of time, and I was continuously upset with my weight. I tried different diets but nothing worked. Exercising was difficult – I would punish myself by going hard at it, but my body couldn't cope. My turning point came when I was getting out of my car one day and it was an effort. I cried and cried. I couldn't stand it anymore and wanted professional help.

I knew when I went to see Arlene that I would have to stop using food to cope. I was sick of hurting my body and feeling ugly and depressed. I found Arlene to be supportive, understanding and sensible in her approach. There was nothing faddish, ridiculous or extreme in her plan. She encouraged me to exercise by simply walking for 45 minutes each day. I live near the beach and found myself reconnecting with nature through these walks. When I saw her plan I realised I'd never been taught how to eat properly. I come from an Italian background where food is closely related to the heart and family, and I had to break away from using food as an emotional crutch. As I ate properly and exercised more the weight began to drop off and my body shape changed. The rolls of fat disappeared from my stomach and I got my waist and curves back.

There were, and still are, times when I fall down and start to slip, but these are becoming rarer. One of my biggest lessons has been not to feel ashamed when I crash, and to ask for help.

So far I've lost 15 kilograms and feel stronger than ever. The best change has been my opinion of myself; my depression has lifted and I am the happiest I've ever been. This is not just because of the external changes in my body; I have a level of self-love and self-respect that I've never had before. I'm not beating myself up with food anymore, and I rarely drink. I eat food with pleasure and in the right way. As a bonus, I receive many compliments about my looks and I'm comfortable with that now. I'm also learning to stand up for myself and figure out what I want in life.

CHAPTER **6**

THE SECOND COMMANDMENT:

Get organised

This is a fundamental commandment, on which all the other commandments depend. If you are not organised, you will have great difficulty gaining control over your eating and exercise – and any other aspects of your life causing you concern. Organisation assists you in balancing your life so you can achieve the harmony you need to succeed.

People are often supremely organised in one aspect of their life – perhaps their job, because their livelihood depends on it – but let everything else slip. They will have the most meticulous files and orderly work procedures, but when it comes to something as basic and important as nourishing themselves, they are in chaos. They have no idea what they will eat from one meal to the next. Consequently, their eating patterns and food intake are inadequate and unacceptable.

Some businesses employ an inventory system called 'just in time': instead of stockpiling components or other supplies necessary to their operations, they order them at the last possible moment, 'just in time'. This might work in an office or factory, but it does not work on the home front, particularly when it comes to enjoying a healthy eating and lifestyle plan. Failure to organise and plan your food supplies results in last-minute panic buying – do you often rush into the supermarket or takeaway after work, when you are tired, crabby and hungry, and grab just about anything that passes as a meal, provided it is quick and easy? You're not alone.

PLANNING AHEAD

The irony is that you could save a lot of time, and eat better, if you planned ahead. It does not take much time and effort, but there are many benefits in terms of caring for yourself.

I have to be extremely organised. My life is very full and busy, because I run my business and am raising two sons. I plan every day to ensure everything runs smoothly. This involves taking care of details. On Monday I have a free hour between 3 p.m. and 4 p.m. to do my shopping for the week. I make a list, head for the supermarket and pick up all the items on my list – I've got my family's meals organised for the week – apart from purchasing the occasional carton of milk and loaf of bread. It takes me an hour to make my shopping list, because I am accustomed to planning meals in advance. This is an essential habit.

WHAT'S FOR DINNER?

Take a few minutes each morning to determine your priorities for the day, starting with planning your meals. When life is hectic it is essential to do this. If you know what your next meal will be – and you have bought the necessary ingredients and might even have already prepared it – you will be better able to resist the impulse to binge when hunger strikes.

Planning your meals does not mean only today's meals, rather everything you will be eating for the entire week. You must sit down with a pen and paper and work out an outline for meals and snacks in advance. This will take time until you are accustomed to doing it, then it will become second nature, like it is for me. (Turn to Chapter 16 for a series of suggested weekly meal plans to help structure your eating and organise your meals.)

Do not be daunted by the thought of planning. Let's put it in perspective. You could easily plan what you are going to wear for the week ahead; you probably organise your holidays months ahead; you plan your children's education years ahead and work out your finances and career path possibly decades ahead. So it is not much of a stretch to plan your meals seven days in advance! Considering our hectic lifestyles, it is essential to pre-organise. The occasional spur-of-the-moment meal is normal and acceptable but will create unnecessary stress if it occurs too often.

SHOP RIGHT

When you have planned the week's meals, you have to shop for the necessary ingredients. People are so busy nowadays that daily food shopping is not always feasible; you might find, as I do, that scheduling an hour at the supermarket once a week is the most effective use of limited time.

Make a list of everything you need before you set out (see the box below for a sample shopping list to get you started). This is an efficient and economical approach, because you are less likely to succumb to unwise impulse purchases. If possible, schedule your shopping expedition on the weekend when you are not stressed or tired. Never shop when you are hungry – it will only make it harder to avoid giving in to temptation.

An alternative is to shop online – many supermarkets offer this service – with groceries ordered on your computer at your convenience and delivered to your door.

Your shopping list

Here is a list of common food items to help you plan your shopping. Why not photocopy this list and use it every time you plan a visit to the supermarket?

Fruit and vegetables

- ☐ apples
- ☐ artichokes
- ☐ apricots
- ☐ asian greens
- ☐ bananas
- ☐ beans (broad, green, string, French)
- ☐ berries (strawberries, blueberries, raspberries, gooseberries)
- ☐ broccoli
- ☐ cabbage (savoy, red)
- ☐ carrots
- ☐ cauliflower
- ☐ celeriac
- ☐ celery
- ☐ cherries
- ☐ corn
- ☐ cucumbers (pickled/ canned/fresh)
- ☐ eggplant

- ☐ garlic
- ☐ ginger
- ☐ grapes
- ☐ lemons
- ☐ lettuce (iceberg, butter, radicchio)
- ☐ limes
- ☐ mangoes
- ☐ melon (watermelon, rockmelon, honeydew)
- ☐ mushrooms
- ☐ nectarines
- ☐ onions (brown, red, spring)
- ☐ oranges
- ☐ peas
- ☐ pears
- ☐ peaches
- ☐ pineapple
- ☐ potatoes
- ☐ pumpkin
- ☐ tomatoes
- ☐ zucchini
- ☐ (other) _____
- ☐ _____
- ☐ _____
- ☐ _____
- ☐ _____
- ☐ _____
- ☐ _____
- ☐ _____
- ☐ _____

Meat and poultry

- ☐ beef (steak, mince, cubed, stir-fry)
- ☐ chicken (breast, stir-fry, mince)
- ☐ eggs
- ☐ lamb
- ☐ pork
- ☐ sausages
- ☐ spatchcock
- ☐ turkey
- ☐ quail
- ☐ (other) _____
- ☐ _____
- ☐ _____
- ☐ _____
- ☐ _____
- ☐ _____
- ☐ _____
- ☐ _____

Fish and seafood

- ☐ barramundi
- ☐ bream
- ☐ calamari
- ☐ cod
- ☐ flake
- ☐ john dory
- ☐ leatherjacket
- ☐ mussels
- ☐ octopus
- ☐ oysters

- ☐ salmon (canned/fresh/ frozen)
- ☐ sardines (canned/fresh)
- ☐ squid
- ☐ swordfish
- ☐ trout
- ☐ tuna (canned/fresh)
- ☐ (other) _____
- ☐ _____
- ☐ _____
- ☐ _____
- ☐ _____
- ☐ _____
- ☐ _____
- ☐ _____

Dairy

- ☐ butter
- ☐ cheese (ricotta, cheddar, cottage, fetta)
- ☐ Fruche lite
- ☐ ice-cream
- ☐ margarine
- ☐ milk
- ☐ yoghurt
- ☐ (other) _____
- ☐ _____
- ☐ _____
- ☐ _____
- ☐ _____
- ☐ _____
- ☐ _____
- ☐ _____

Beverages

- ☐ Bonox
- ☐ cocoa
- ☐ coffee
- ☐ cordial
- ☐ Jarrah hot chocolate/ Swiss Miss/Ovaltine Lite/Cadbury Lite
- ☐ mineral water
- ☐ soft drinks (low-joule tonic, ginger beer, cola, lemonade)
- ☐ tea
- ☐ (other) _____
- ☐ _____
- ☐ _____
- ☐ _____
- ☐ _____
- ☐ _____
- ☐ _____
- ☐ _____

Staples

- ☐ breads
- ☐ cereal
- ☐ crispbreads, crackers
- ☐ crumpets, English muffins
- ☐ dried fruit (sultanas, raisins, dried apricots)
- ☐ flour (plain, self-raising, cornflour)
- ☐ noodles

- [ ] nuts (cashews, peanuts, walnuts, pecans, almonds, pistachios)
- [ ] oil (olive, canola, sesame)
- [ ] pasta
- [ ] rice (brown, wild, basmati, jasmine)
- [ ] (other) _____
- [ ] _____
- [ ] _____
- [ ] _____
- [ ] _____
- [ ] _____
- [ ] _____
- [ ] _____

Smallgoods

- [ ] bacon
- [ ] corned beef/rare roast beef
- [ ] ham
- [ ] pastrami
- [ ] (other) _____
- [ ] _____
- [ ] _____
- [ ] _____
- [ ] _____

- [ ] _____
- [ ] _____
- [ ] _____

Condiments

- [ ] chutney
- [ ] curry paste (red, green, yellow)
- [ ] herbs (parsley, rosemary, thyme, mint, coriander, sage)
- [ ] pepper (black, white, pink)
- [ ] salt (table salt, sea salt, rock salt)
- [ ] sauces (hoisin, plum, barbecue, sweet chilli, soy)
- [ ] spices (nutmeg, cinnamon, five spice)
- [ ] (other) _____
- [ ] _____
- [ ] _____
- [ ] _____
- [ ] _____
- [ ] _____
- [ ] _____
- [ ] _____

Also keep a stock of frozen and canned products, which can be used to prepare a quick, easy and tasty meal. Only utilise low-joule frozen pre-cooked meals as a last resort.

KEEP IT CONVENIENT

You should not compromise on the quality of your food; it must be the best you can afford. Try to take advantage of all the conveniences and short cuts available to today's shoppers. Supermarkets now stock salad packs, soup packs and vegetable stir-fries – all washed, chopped and mixed ready for you to cook or serve. Butchers offer trimmed, chopped and marinated cuts of meats. When time is at a premium, these short cuts help you make healthy food choices – you only have to control portion size.

Are you too busy to cook during the working week? Set aside a morning on the weekend to shop and prepare meals – such as casseroles, soups and curries – you can enjoy the entire week. Do you spend a lot of time on the road? Devise coping strategies that suit your schedule: go online before leaving home to check out healthy restaurants at your destination or pre-pack meals in a cooler bag. Your eating is too important to leave to chance.

GET IN EARLY

To get organised you must identify times that are going to be difficult to cope, when it is easy to sabotage your efforts. Six o'clock can be a very stressful time. Rushing home from work, picking up children from school or long day care – everybody is tired and hungry. This is not the time to have to wait for food or to spend a lot of time preparing dinner.

Rather than attempting to make an elaborate dinner from scratch (or pick up a takeaway), get up 20 minutes earlier in the morning and make a salad, chop the vegetables, prepare a curry, casserole or other dish that you can get ready ahead of time. Everything is organised, so when you arrive home that night all you have to do is pop the meat and vegetables in the oven, lay the table and you're ready to eat.

Another great strategy is to invest in a slow cooker, in which you put the makings of the meal (anything from soup to a whole chicken) in the morning, and arrive home at night to a feast cooked to perfection. Barbecues and stir-fries are also delicious, quick, low-fat cooking methods.

REASSESS THE CONTENTS OF YOUR KITCHEN

Your kitchen is the epicentre of your efforts to lose weight. Stocking the correct items in the required amounts will prevent you from undermining your best intentions. Review your food supply. Check out the pantry and refrigerator and remove anything you are likely to binge on. We tend to eat what is most available, and if that is junk (high in saturated fat and sugar, and low in fibre), that is what we will eat. If healthier choices are accessible, we will consume those. Stock your refrigerator and cupboards with a healthy selection every week.

Organise a good workspace and ensure that all the utensils you need to prepare meals are close to hand. You should always have the basics to enable you to cook a quick and nutritious meal at any time. The knowledge that you can do this helps allay the anxiety over what you can prepare, and how quickly the food can be on the table.

STRUCTURING YOUR LIFE

The importance of structure applies to every aspect of your life, not just your eating. Take exercise, for example. An early riser will exercise in the early hours of the morning, whereas a late riser might prefer to do an exercise session at lunchtime or in the evening. You have to schedule your activities to best suit your life patterns and biorhythms – everyone is

Managing your time

This much-discussed art is the bedrock of organising your eating and other important aspects of your life. Volumes have been written on this topic, however exploring it in detail is beyond the scope of this book. Here are a few tips for you to consider.

- Make a list of everything you want to achieve each day.
- Assign a priority to each task, and tackle the high-priority tasks first.
- Do it – now!
- Tick off tasks as you accomplish them; this will add to your sense of achievement.
- Learn to delegate to others – you don't have to do everything yourself.
- Regularly review your program to consider which tasks are essential and which could be dropped. Filling your day with pointless activity only increases stress and fatigue – enemies of sensible eating!

different and there are no strict rules, provided you form a structure that you find acceptable.

Most people are time-short and try to do a lot in their day. If you don't manage your time – down to working out when you're going to exercise and arrange your meals – you could well have difficulty coping with your weight loss and a weight maintenance regime.

START NOW

If you have not previously thought about structuring your shopping, cooking and eating, and you think you might find it difficult, do not despair. You are almost certainly a more organised person than you realise. Everybody has some form of structure in their life. If you are working, you probably keep a diary of your appointments to organise your day. By doing this you are structuring your work life.

You must take the same approach when structuring your eating plan. If you have a 2 p.m. appointment, you must eat your lunch before, so plan for that. Will you make lunch in the morning before leaving for work? If not, will you have the time to buy it before the appointment? And, more importantly, will you have time to sit and eat it?

Planning is essential. Typically you would rush to that appointment with no time to eat; you might grab a muffin at a convenience store along the way. Now, muffins are not particularly nourishing and are loaded in kilojoules, and yet you probably won't feel as though you have eaten because you had it on the run. If you really wanted that muffin, fine – you should have sat down and enjoyed it. Grabbing it might make you feel that you have blown your day. This could trigger a binge, which is due primarily to lack of preparation.

One day of your life is inconsequential, but if every day is like this, it will result in a weight problem ... and a lot of unnecessary distress. In addition, you are not establishing good habits that make you feel better, more in control and able to deal with life's hurdles. Organising your life, eating and exercise is not difficult, it just requires planning, the same way every aspect of life needs to be balanced and prioritised.

> *'Whether you think you can or think you can't, you're right'*
>
> HENRY FORD

CRISIS PLANNING

Ever had one of those days when everything seems to go wrong and the only thing that is going to make you feel better is a great big piece of chocolate cake or a packet of chips? You are normal. There is nothing accidental about those bad days, and it is not really an impulse decision to eat that cake. In fact, most people know when they wake up in the morning which days are going to be a struggle – it could be due to biorhythms, but it's generally an emotional state – and they have a pretty good idea that they are going to be indulging in some comfort eating.

Fatigue is often the initiator. Thursdays I always struggle.

I start work early, work a long day and then I am busy with the children after work. Plan for those days. Program that piece of chocolate cake into your weekly eating so that you can enjoy it without worrying that you've blown it or failed.

Group support

Question: My co-workers and I are starting a diet support club. Our ages vary from 18 to 70, and we have different dietary requirements and weight goals. How can we coordinate everyone's needs and preferences?

Answer: Congratulations – you are starting by organising yourselves, which is the essential first step. Pick an end point – three months away, for example – and schedule weekly meetings. At the first meeting, have everyone write down their nutrition and exercise goals. Do not focus on weight but on developing healthy eating habits, because this is the key to success. Weigh yourselves and take your measurements, because this is often a better gauge than a scale. During the three months everybody should aim to make a few changes, such as omitting butter, margarine and mayonnaise; consuming smaller portions of lollies and chocolates; and refusing second helpings. Similarly make your exercise goals specific, realistic and measurable. Log your progress, and write down a reward for attaining each goal – anything that makes you feel good, as long as it is not food! Share your experiences, positive and negative, with your diet buddies; often others can see your success when you cannot, or can come up with solutions to obstacles you are facing. The group support will motivate you to maintain good habits!

Getting organised does not happen immediately. Perseverance eventually leads to habits being developed. Everything in life requires hard work and practice before habits are altered and become second nature, and not a chore.

Occasionally unexpected situations arise – you get stuck in traffic, you get called to the school because your child is sick – and your well-prepared plans are forfeited, c'est la vie! There is a difference between the occasional deviation from a plan, and never having one to begin with.

There is nothing spontaneous about losing weight – it is continual hard work! You have to show discipline, determination and organisation. But if you follow my advice, you can do it!

Putting the steam back into your self-esteem

It's not just your work diary or your kitchen cupboards that you have to reorganise; it could also be your approach to losing weight, and indeed to yourself. I'm referring to your self-esteem, which could be defined as unconditional self-acceptance and self-respect. A healthy level of self-esteem is essential for you to be able to effectively function, both personally and professionally. You have to believe you can do something to be successful!

How can you turn low self-esteem around and avoid a vicious cycle of self-destruction?

- Stop putting yourself down. Whenever you have a negative thought like, 'I'm hopeless, I'll always be fat,' replace it with a self-respectful, positive thought, such as, 'I haven't lost as much weight as I would have liked to date, but that does not mean I never will. Slow weight loss is acceptable, and the beginning of the path to my actual goal.'

- Identify the cause of your previous failure, and ways you can rectify it. You have replaced feelings of failure with an action plan.

- Recognise your achievements – acknowledge that you are a competent, worthwhile person.

- Create a list of your positive attributes.

- Consistently make small changes, and eventually you will notice their impact on your weight, health, energy level and even your mood!

- Be aware that big changes, such as losing a lot of weight, can be scary and intimidating. It is normal to feel daunted from time to time. Change takes time to adapt to, and courage to accept. Be prepared to forgive yourself your failures, as long as you keep on trying. Do not give up on yourself!

SUMMING UP

* Have faith in yourself. If you can organise your work or family life, you can organise a packed lunch and prepare dinner in advance.

* Make time for shopping and cooking (and, of course, eating, because there is no point in making a delicious dinner if you don't give yourself the time to appreciate it).

* Plan ahead so that you are never frenetically hungry – you know when to expect your next meal.

* Anticipate bad days and structure them into your eating plan.

* When you are organised you will be less fatigued and anxious, so you will be able to relax, enjoy your meal and feel satisfied with smaller portions.

SUCCESS *Max* STORY

I migrated to Australia in April 2000. I had always been fit, spent a lot of time in the gym and managed to maintain a weight of 83 kilograms. As I tried to settle into a new country, my time for exercise was limited, and my weight began to increase because I ate out a lot. After a while I weighed 99 kilograms and was feeling sick and uncomfortable. I was introduced to Arlene and started visiting her on a weekly basis. Arlene stressed that I had to get my life together; I had to start eating properly, exercising regularly and become positive in all respects. I began following Arlene's eating plan and started walking 10 000 steps every day. I achieved my goal weight of 83 kilograms, and my weight has remained constant for the past two years. I still follow Arlene's advice. I eat what I like, but in moderation. I exercise at least five days a week, and I am thrilled with my new lifestyle. I feel healthy, confident and successful, and I have a sense of control over my food and my life.

CHAPTER 7

THE THIRD COMMANDMENT:

Eat small

People often ask me how many kilojoules they should consume each day, and I always tell them I don't want them to
think in terms of kilojoules, because this only contributes to
the sense of 'being on a diet', rather than adopting a healthy
lifetime eating plan. Keeping an eye on the size of the portions of your food is more crucial.

Consider what is on your plate; not just the type of food,
but also the quantity of it. You
might be surprised to learn
how much you are eating in
a 'normal' meal – it could be a
great deal more than you realise. Have you ever felt that you
were doing everything correctly
in terms of eating and exercising, and still you couldn't shed
the excess kilos ... or even put

> 'The road to
> success is dotted
> with many
> tempting parking
> places'
>
> ——
>
> ANON.

on weight? So what is going wrong?

You have been eating more than your body needs. Often, much more. Overweight people consistently underestimate how much they eat at a sitting, while underweight people overestimate the amount. The bottom line is portion size. I often send new clients to a nearby cafe to buy a sandwich that I know will be a generous size. Underweight people (yes, people who need to put *on* weight consult me as well as people who want to lose it) invariably say that they can't possibly finish the sandwich. The overweight people consume the entire sandwich and then feel satisfied that all they have had for lunch was a single sandwich – not realising that portion sizes – which we accept as average – are larger than they have ever been.

In Australia portions tend to be large, and are getting larger, which is why portion control is so crucial to reaching and maintaining a healthy weight. This can be quite hard to do in this supersize age, in which cafe and restaurant meals are often big enough to feed two or more people, and snacks and prepared foods come in jumbo sizes and value packs. Consider how muffins have ballooned over the past few years; once they were the size of a cupcake, now they're huge, more than double their original dimensions. Yet because the normal tendency is to eat what's in front of us, we consume the entire serving, sometimes returning for seconds.

Consider children who eat only as much as they need. They seldom finish what is given to them – if you give them a sandwich, they may only eat part of it. And they adjust their

Too much of a good thing

Question: Since commencing a secretarial job, my weight has increased rapidly. I eat very lightly – toast and a cup of tea for breakfast, a tuna-and-salad sandwich for lunch, and yoghurt and a muesli bar in the afternoon. For dinner I normally have pasta, fish and vegetables or baked beans, or other healthy foods. So why the sudden increase?

Answer: Despite how 'healthy' a food might be, you can still eat too much of it, and it appears as though this is what is causing your weight gain. Weight loss works on the simple equation of energy in versus energy out. You are obviously taking in too many kilojoules for your activity level, so be aware of your portion sizes. A sedentary job doesn't help, so try to include at least 45 minutes of aerobic exercise in your day. If you are exercising and consuming the correct-sized portions of the foods you describe, your weight will definitely begin to drop.

intake to their activity level. If they're playing a lot of sport, they will eat more to fuel the extra energy utilised while exercising, but when they're less active – studying for an exam, playing on the computer or reading – they will eat less.

Many adults have lost the ability to do this. Perhaps it is because we've been brought up to finish what is on our plate, and to think of the 'starving children in Africa or India'. Unfortunately, overeating destroys the natural instinct the body has of indicating how much we should eat and when we are comfortably full, resulting in us getting fatter. These ingrained habits persist, whatever the size of the serving. As the servings in Australia have grown, we have become accustomed to eating more.

PETITE PORTIONS KEEP THE FRENCH SLIM

Compare the way we eat here with the way people eat in France. The French are famed for their cuisine. The food is delicious, and not exactly low-fat, often with cream, butter and brandy. This is, after all, the nation that invented *pâté de foie gras*. So why are only 10 per cent of French people overweight or obese, compared with over 30 per cent of Australians? The answer has a lot to do with portion sizes.

In an elegant piece of scientific detection, researchers weighed portions at restaurants in Sydney and Paris and also checked common food items sold in supermarkets in both countries. From confectionery through to takeaway items, the serving sizes were consistently much larger in Australia than in France. For example, an order of (yes, French) fries here was 48 per cent larger; a single chocolate was 41 per cent larger; a soft drink was 52 per cent larger; a pot of yoghurt was 50 per cent larger and a Chinese restaurant meal was a whopping 70 per cent larger.

Even at expensive restaurants in France, the servings are small; they believe in giving you tiny tastes of a variety of dishes, not a mountain of two or three items, as we do in Australia. You might think that such tiny tastes would only whet your appetite but, in fact, they are quite satisfying. If you eat slowly and savour every mouthful when everything is so delicious, you don't need large quantities.

How you view mealtime can also affect the amount of food you eat. The French see meals as opportunities for relaxing social occasions rather than as a rush to consume a meal in as short a time as possible, as we tend to do here – we are always in a hurry. Eating should never be rushed or uncontrolled, because this leads to overeating. Even at fast-food restaurants, the French spend more time at the table

Think thin

An important step to effective long-term weight loss is to start thinking like a thin person. How do thin people think and behave? They eat when they are hungry and stop when their appetite is satisfied. They enjoy their food and eat what they like – often the same foods that you love and crave – but the big difference is that the portions they eat are typically small. They opt for quality, not quantity: a morsel of a really good cheese rather than a big lump of the rubbery, low-fat, processed variety. They appreciate and taste their food – something we should all do, because eating is one of life's great pleasures – maximising enjoyment, not kilojoules. Make everything you eat the best quality you can afford, because when the focus is on taste, rather than amount, you're less likely to overeat.

than Australians – an average of 22 minutes versus 14 minutes – in addition to eating a lot less in this time. This translates to putting time aside to enjoy your meal and relish every mouthful, which is how I would like you to approach your meals in the future.

MAKE A FIST OF IT

How big *should* your portions be? Here's a handy rule of thumb: when it comes to a meal, the carbohydrate (such as couscous, rice, pasta or potato) and protein (such as meat, chicken or fish) portions on your plate should each not be any larger than the size of your clenched fist; so that's a fist of carbohydrate and a fist of protein. Consider that the average serving is often two or three times larger than that; this might not seem much for an entire meal. If I sat down with you and showed you the size of the portions you should be having, as opposed to what you're probably eating now, you wouldn't believe your eyes.

Your stomach is a muscle that is roughly the size of your fist, and this amount fills it nicely. Many of us continually stretch and overstretch our stomach by eating huge portions at a sitting, which is why the capacity of the stomach of an overweight or obese person has been shown to be much larger than that of a lean person. Your stomach will take time to return to its normal size. You will be hungry for a few weeks as your system adjusts to your new regime of smaller portions. That thought should not make you feel anxious, because downsizing your portions will eventually come to feel normal as you learn to eat until you are comfortable, never till you are bloated or full.

EATING IN

Eating out has become very popular and common. It could be for the convenience, it could be to save time, it could be the best way for us to socialise with family and friends, or it could be because we don't enjoy cooking. This is a pity,

Jane, 22, office manager

Jane eats her food very quickly; a bad habit she is trying to break because she finishes her meal when her friends have just started eating. She will then have second helpings to keep them company. 'My parents ate very quickly, so we kids grew up following suit,' she explains. 'It didn't help that you had to finish what was on your plate before you could have dessert, so the first person to finish the main course got the most sweets.' Mealtimes became a race between Jane and her three siblings; it was a case of first in, best dressed, and they would pile their dessert bowls high. Eating too much too quickly becomes a habit over time. 'Our portions were pretty big,' she admits. 'Now I tell myself: take your time, put a little on your plate, eat it slowly and then see how hungry you're feeling before you have more.' Remember that it takes twenty minutes for your brain to get the message from your stomach that it has had something to eat.

because it means that we are handing control over what we eat to commercial operators whose focus is on controlling costs, not kilojoules. Bulking up mass-produced meals with cheap ingredients such as fat and sugar is one way to do that, which is why a typical takeaway meal will set you back 4200–6720 kilojoules versus 2520–2940 kilojoules for a healthy home-cooked meal. Ingredients aside, the size of takeaway and restaurant meals are usually generous to a fault, which can play havoc with your efforts to control portion sizes.

I would like you to make a resolution to cook and eat at home as often as you can. Start with the most important meal of the day – breakfast. People who eat at home, especially breakfast, are the most successful at losing weight and keeping it off, because they're less likely to binge later in the day. Home cooking also helps you regain control over your food intake, allowing you to save hundreds of kilojoules and loads of fat per meal. Cooking for yourself allows you to prepare food the way you want it – roasted on a rack, for example, rather than deep-fried. Shopping for ingredients and cooking your own meals means you can select the best-quality ingredients, and you are more likely to control your portions sizes and save leftovers for later. In a restaurant you might feel too shy to ask for a doggie bag, and so you might eat the lot on the spot.

No time to cook? Make time. You can whip up a healthy meal, such as an omelette with asparagus on the side, with virtually no fat in a non-stick pan, in 10 minutes – the time that you would waste waiting for a takeaway. Another advantage of taking the time at home is the difference in nutrition content in your homemade meal. An egg-white omelette always looks like a good alternative when you eat out – as it is at home. However, when you see the chef generously ladle a clear liquid into the pan before making your favourite, you should know that the liquid is fat, and the ladle holds at least 2 tablespoons. That is 22 grams of fat, mostly saturated fat (16 grams), and another 840 kilojoules to your so-called 'healthy' dish. A good reason to eat at home!

Everyone is a chef in the making

You think you don't know how to cook? That was the case for Jonathan, a teacher who was so tired after a day in front of the classroom that he usually bought takeaway on his way home. Jonathan, 32, was single and didn't enjoy eating alone, so he would turn on the television for company. This resulted in him eating more than he realised, because he was so preoccupied with his favourite shows he wasn't keeping track of his intake over the course of an evening in front of the box. Even though Jonathan knew his weight was increasing, he found it hard to break the takeaway habit, because he wasn't confident in the kitchen; in fact, he'd hardly ever done more than make a sandwich or boil an egg. Then Jonathan spotted a brochure for the local night school, which was offering Chinese-cooking classes. He signed up, and found that not only did he learn to cook his favourite cuisine, but, because the class would end with the students consuming their creations, he was eating with company and making new friends. 'It's a lot of fun – sort of like a low-stress dinner party every week,' says Jonathan, who's gone on to take classes in Italian and Thai cooking, and has tried out many of the recipes at home for himself. Many busy people in the workforce are in Jonathan's situation; if you're one of them and have never really learned to cook, why not invest in a few classes? Look in your local paper or search the Internet and you will discover great cooking courses available for varying levels of cooking and different cuisines.

You don't need to be a great cook to eat well. Grilling or barbecuing a steak or fillet of fish and serving it with a fresh garden salad, with fruit to follow, is well within the capacity of any novice, and it still tastes delicious and takes very little time to prepare. Why eat out when you can dine like a king at home – and save on both money and kilojoules!

EATING OUT

There will be times when you want – or are obliged – to eat out. Business often involves breakfast meetings, working lunches and dinners with clients. And you should not refuse friends if they ask you to join them for a restaurant meal. You do not have to restrict your social life to lose weight, because it is all part of adapting to a new lifestyle – the choices you make and the portions you eat.

Settle for halves

Restaurants often dish up enormous servings, and many people find it difficult to leave anything on their plate,

Four ways to downsize dinner

1. Buy only as much as you plan to consume at a sitting; for example, a mini-roast, which you can buy at many butchers nowadays, rather than an entire leg of lamb. Sure, you'll have leftovers for later if you invest in the latter . . . but you're more likely to eat more when there are second helpings of an appetising roast in front of you.

2. Serve your meal on a smaller plate – entree size rather than main size. Your plate will look satisfyingly full with considerably less food.

3. Dish up meals in the kitchen, never from a platter or pot placed on the table, because having extra food in front of you only encourages picking extras from the pot.

4. As soon as you have cooked and served your meal, put away all unused portions; freezing leftovers immediately is a safe way of ensuring that you don't go back for seconds.

especially when they're paying for it. Ideally order an entree size, or share a main meal between two. Many restaurants and cafes will give you smaller servings if you ask. A man I know has a deal with a restaurant where he regularly dines: he pays the full price but they serve him half-portions. Consequently, he never sees what he's missing and is perfectly happy consuming less.

Plan ahead

Remember how southern belles managed to maintain a 'ladylike' – meaning small – appetite in Margaret Mitchell's classic novel *Gone with the Wind*? They ate before going out, in order to not need to touch the feast on offer at parties and balls. Like them, why not have a light snack in the late afternoon – such as fruit, salad, soup or yoghurt – to take the edge off your appetite, before going to the restaurant?

Once out, commence with a non-alcoholic drink (sparkling water or lime-and-soda is ideal, but in the cold weather this could be a cappuccino or tea); this will help to fill you up, and slow you down when the food arrives. It can also be a 'filler' while everyone is munching on snacks or bread. Go slow on the alcohol, because it weakens your willpower. Try not to have more than two alcoholic drinks at a sitting, otherwise you will probably eat more than you intended to. (More about alcohol on page 164.) Oh, and never butter your bread, because it can make even the stalest roll palatable. Ideally, give the bread a miss completely!

For more on wise choices when eating in restaurants, turn to Chapter 17 for the lowdown on popular cuisines.

EATING AT A FRIEND'S HOUSE

Nothing is nicer than being entertained in the home of friends. In terms of your eating plan, however, this is trickier than eating at a restaurant because you have no say over what is served, how it is prepared or when it will be served. The conflict between good manners and your desire to adhere to your new eating plan can blow your best intentions.

Don't fret – with a little forethought you can enjoy social-ising with friends while still eating normally. Eat a snack before you leave home to take the edge off your hunger and to sustain you if dinner is served late. Request small portions so you do not overeat. And remember, it is not bad manners to leave something on your plate.

If your hosts have spent hours toiling in the kitchen mak-ing a feast for you and your fellow guests, eat small quantities of what they have prepared, because it would be rude not to. However, this only applies to what they have made them-selves, as Marianne, a publicist with a very active social life, has discovered. 'I make a point of only eating what someone has personally cooked, not food they have bought, because the home-cooked stuff is what they've really invested in emo-tionally,' she explains. 'They're not going to be offended or even notice if I pass on things like pre-dinner nibbles, bread rolls, cheese or after-dinner mints.' You never have to eat until you are full, and you are entitled to inform your host that you appreciate all the trouble they have gone to in preparing such a delicious meal, but you cannot eat anything more – just a teaspoon taste because you don't want to miss out!

Be lavish with your praise and they are unlikely to notice the quantities you have eaten. Above all, resist the temptation to announce to all present that you are watching your weight. They will all groan. It is not a diet; your weight will drop from adopting new habits and eating more carefully – even when out to dinner or entertaining.

If you do slip up and lash out, don't despair. The occasional blowout isn't going to derail your new eating plan. As Scarlett O'Hara used to say, tomorrow is another day. Try to be careful with your food choices and increase your exercise the next day and you will feel better and more motivated to adhere to a healthy regime.

Taming your appetite

It's all very well to talk about small portions and tiny tastes, but sometimes your appetite feels like a ravenous beast. It doesn't care about your figure or your health. How to tame this wild animal? Don't try to defeat it; satisfy it.

Many people enjoy the feeling of being 'full'; when they are unable to eat another bite. But you do not have to gorge yourself on high-fat, energy-dense food to feel full. Scientists have discovered that people tend to eat around the same amount of food every day, regardless of how many kilojoules or how much fat, protein or carbohydrate it contains. It is mostly volume – the simple mass of food that you consume, not the type of food – that produces that feeling of your appetite being satisfied. This means you can eat quite a lot of low-energy-dense food – foods that fill you up but are relatively low in kilojoules – and satisfy your appetite without gaining weight.

So what are these low-energy, high-volume, appetite-busting substances? You'll be surprised how familiar and tasty they are.

Soup

This old favourite satisfies almost every sense. Your eyes see a generous volume. The delicious aroma delights your nose. The large amount of liquid (mostly water) quickly fills your stomach. The ingredients – vegetables and tasty herbs – take time to digest, helping to make you feel satisfied for longer. Chewy soups with plenty of substance – containing beans, lentils, whole grains and the like – are excellent choices. Be wary of cream-based soups, because they are high in fat and consequently kilojoules. Soup is an excellent starter, and because it is so hearty you'll eat less for subsequent courses. If you don't feel like hot soup, start with a glass of vegetable juice; this is also very satisfying and filling. In the summer there are many cold soups that are nutritious and delicious, such as Gazpacho, beetroot and chilled tomato.

Tuna

Protein is more filling, bite for bite, than fat. Fish produces a great sense of fullness, so opt for tuna, sardines or salmon (if you're choosing the canned variety opt for fish packed in brine, not oil), because they are rich in healthy omega-3 fatty acids.

Low-fat milk

Believe it or not, drinking milk before or during a meal helps you feel full quickly and you tend to eat less at your next meal. Paradoxically, the lighter the milk, the greater the effect, because you can fill up on more light milk for fewer kilojoules.

Berries

Sweet and juicy, berries and other fruits make the smartest and most delicious snacks of all. Along with high water content, berries are high in fibre, so fill you up with few kilojoules.

Compare these three snacks: 2¾ cups of strawberries; 18 fat-free pretzels; 10 jelly beans. Each contains approximately 420 kilojoules, but the strawberries are much more likely to curb your appetite than the pretzels or jelly beans because the volume is far greater.

Rice

Rice is a staple of cultures that have traditionally been lean for millennia. That is because rice satisfies you for relatively few kilojoules. Try this for a filling Chinese meal: 120 grams chicken, 1½ cups broccoli in hoisin sauce and ⅔ cup cooked rice. All that, for just 1680 kilojoules!

Frozen desserts

Can't enjoy dinner without dessert? Relax, it needn't be fattening. A frozen dessert – an icy pole, some frozen yoghurt, a scoop of low-fat ice-cream or gelato – is a great way to satisfy your sweet tooth without overdoing it.

Bran flakes

These aren't just a terrific source of fibre, they take the edge off your appetite for longer than many other foods at the cost of very few kilojoules. Add bran flakes to bulk up your breakfast cereal, fruit or low-fat yoghurt.

Fruit smoothies

Reach for the blender and make a smoothie of ½ banana, ½ cup frozen strawberries and 1 cup milk. This has a good balance of all your nutrients, including vitamins and minerals.

In general, discover the satisfying tastes of fruits, vegetables, bread and cereals that have bulk and are filling without providing excess kilojoules.

SUMMING UP

* Watch your portion sizes.
* Know your appetite. The moment that you feel comfortably full, stop eating. It is an elementary but very effective weight-control skill – stop when your stomach has had enough!
* Cook for yourself and try to eat at home as often as possible.
* Plan ahead when you do eat out. Make sure you don't arrive hungry, and work out ways to reduce eating the quantities of food on offer.

SUCCESS STORY
Susanne

I have always had a weight problem. I came from a Jewish family where food was always around in generous quantities. I was never encouraged to lose weight, even though I tried every new fad diet and failed. We always had very good food at home; no junk food. I just ate too much. I was a yo-yo dieter, losing 5 kilograms and then putting on 6 kilograms. When I got married I weighed 64 kilograms; by the time I was in my late thirties and early forties I weighed 76 kilograms. I tried many diets promising quick and easy results – and I always failed, which made me very unhappy. I finally came to realise that losing weight and keeping it off is not quick and easy. I made a decision to go and see a dietician to help me achieve permanent weight loss.

Arlene helped me to understand that I was eating too much. I had to learn to eat much smaller portions. I also came to understand that I was an emotional eater. I would medicate myself with food in response to guilt, stress and anger or positive emotions such as happiness and joy.

I had to change my environment and make it fail-proof. I had to learn new behaviours – never leave a meal feeling full; walk every day; eat three meals a day; have two small snacks; never go shopping for food when hungry; and remember to be nice to yourself every day!

I realised that this is not a diet; this is a way of life. It took me at least two years to lose the weight. I lost 15 kilograms – that was four years ago. I continue to see Arlene because I know I have the type of personality that needs to be accountable to someone other than myself.

Losing the weight took me a long time, and keeping it off is hard work. But one thing I know – the payoff is great! I feel good and I am very healthy. Shopping for clothes is fun!

CHAPTER **8**

THE FOURTH COMMANDMENT:

Learn to leave food on your plate

Do you remember when you were young and your grand-mother told you it was good manners to leave something on your plate? Confusingly, this instruction conflicted with the other traditional mealtime admonition: Finish what's on your plate or there will be no dessert. No wonder you ended up completely baffled!

Like so much folk wisdom, this first instruction has a kernel of wisdom in it . . . which is why this is my fourth commandment: Learn to leave food on your plate. This old-fashioned virtue is the key to controlling your eating. It's all part of training yourself to see food differently – as something to be savoured and enjoyed, not to be consumed in a frenzy.

Consequently, with every meal remind yourself that you don't have to clean your plate. If you have your meals organised correctly and eat three snacks each day, you will not be ravenously hungry, and you will feel comfortable about when your next meal/snack is being eaten. You can therefore quite contentedly leave something on your plate. Why? It's a symbolic act. By choosing to leave a little on your plate, you are proving to yourself that you are in control of your food; it does not control you. You prefer not to binge; you decide to eat the correct amount to meet your physical needs as you attain a healthy weight. To demonstrate this, you choose to leave a little behind.

How much food should you leave on your plate? It doesn't really matter. Improved eating habits are a discipline that I would like you to learn; they have nothing to do with the number of kilojoules you consumed in a meal. So, I don't care if you leave just a mouthful of food or half your

A matter of choice

Some people blame their parents for the fact that they always polish their plate, never leaving a bite of food. It is, they say, the way most of us were conditioned, and it is too difficult to change. Some parents do encourage their children to overeat, and it is difficult to change bad habits, but it *can* be done, and it must be if you want to control your eating. Now is the time for you to take responsibility for your weight problems. You cannot keep thinking about the past if you want to start living your future and enjoying every day without the constant worry about food, eating, weight and dieting.

dinner, I want you to get over the old pattern of finishing everything on your plate. Just leave something, to show you are in control. Ideally eat until you are comfortable, never until you are full.

> '*I can resist everything except temptation*'
>
> OSCAR WILDE

What do you do with the remains on the plate? Remove them immediately – either by throwing them out or storing them in a container in the fridge. In a restaurant ask the waiter to take away your plate. If you sit looking at the leftovers, you are more likely to eat them. The sight of food is a cue to eat – even a few scraps on a plate – so don't make life more difficult by putting temptation in front of you.

CUES CONTROL

Everywhere we turn there are cues encouraging us to eat more than we need or even want. We are surrounded by food – at home, in shops, restaurants, the staffroom at work and even vending machines in public places. Magazines and newspapers are full of images of food. Every second television program seems to feature a celebrity chef cooking up a storm, and that's not counting all the food commercials in the ad breaks. Bookshops offer numerous cookbooks, despite the fact that fewer meals are prepared in the home. Our social lives revolve around food – let's do lunch, let's go for coffee, I'll meet you for dinner, pop in for tea and biscuits.

Often these cues are unrelated to hunger. It might simply be the time of day prompting us to eat because that is when we are used to eating, regardless of whether or not we are hungry. We frequently eat because the person we are socialising with is eating. Other cues include appetising aromas and non-food related activities that we have come to associate with eating, such as watching television. (More on this on page 156).

These cues are remarkably powerful. Consider these seven common cues to eat, and strategies to counteract them.

Cue 1: The sight of food

The most powerful stimulus to over-consumption is simply the sight of food – it is difficult to resist temptation when there is something to eat directly in front of you. The more food you see, the more you will probably eat. Hunger or even taste don't seem important – when the food is there, people will eat it until it is finished. When people helped themselves to soup from a trick bowl that never became empty, no matter how much was consumed (it refilled itself from a reservoir hidden under the table), everyone consumed more than their usual portion size simply because there was so much soup available. The sight of soup was the cue to start eating, but the corresponding cue to stop eating – an empty bowl – was absent, so they continued eating.

Solution: Avoid smorgasbords and all-you-can eat meal deals, because these only encourage overeating. Don't go to the supermarket when you are hungry, and don't browse gourmet food shops for fun, because you will probably succumb to buying too liberally. Eat until your hunger is satisfied, never until you are bloated. Fill yourself up with high-fibre, high-water-content foods such as vegetables, salads and soups. Nobody ever got fat from eating large helpings of salad greens! And of course, learn to leave food on your plate.

Cue 2: Availability

If snacks are close at hand, obtainable without any effort, you are likely to pick at them all day. When chocolates and lollies were in view on office desks, workers ate an average of nine pieces a day, and tended to lose track of how many they had eaten. When the sweets were in their drawer, the workers averaged six pieces per day, whereas when the sweets were stored out of sight 6 metres from their desks, the workers ate just four.

Solution: Hide tempting treats and keep snacks out of reach and sight. If you must have something to nibble while you work, make it celery or carrot sticks.

Cue 3: Too many choices

Eating a variety of foods ensures that you will satisfy all your nutrient requirements. However, too much variety can result in overeating – all those tempting choices and flavours. It is a fine balance steering a course between sufficient and excessive variety. When people were presented with three different shapes of pasta, they ate 15 per cent more than when they were given their single favourite shape. Similarly, when offered M&Ms in ten colours, people ate 25–30 per cent more than when they were only offered seven colours.

Solution: Indulge your need for variety with a wide selection of foods that are low in kilojoules but high in flavour, such as fruit, vegetables, legumes, soup and low-fat yoghurt. Fill your plate with salad greens and lots of vegetables first, and then take a small portion of meat/pasta/rice. This way you will feel so satisfied that you will have little appetite for snacking.

Cue 4: Special offers

Most fast-food restaurants offer such great deals on super-sized portions that you feel foolish ordering smaller servings. Most of us can't resist a bargain! The pricing system is all wrong because it encourages over-consumption.

Solution: Be vigilant – those bargain-basement 'meal deals' are only undermining your desire to make good choices in the correct volume! Ask yourself whether getting your money's worth in the form of huge portions is really more important than reaching your goal weight, staying healthy and feeling better.

Cue 5: Optical illusions

People perceive a tall, slender glass as holding more liquid than a short, wide one, even when the two glasses hold the same amount. Our eyes tend to focus on height, causing us to underestimate the volume of the shorter glass. This was illustrated when people poured fruit juice into both types of glasses – they drank nearly 20 per cent more from the short glasses.

Solution: Think tall and skinny. When enjoying high-kilojoule drinks such as fruit juices, smoothies or alcoholic beverages use tall, narrow glasses. You will think that you have drunk more than you actually have, so you will feel satisfied with less.

Cue 6: Misleading labels

Labelling foods as 'low fat', 'reduced fat' or 'lite' is another stimulant for buying. If we perceive that food is less 'fattening', we respond by eating more. First, these terms can be quite misleading (for example, 'low fat' could just mean lower in fat than the regular version of the item in question, not necessarily low in fat in overall terms). Second, eating more of a low-fat item than you would of a higher fat version results in a greater intake of fat and kilojoules . . . so you have achieved nothing!

Solution: Always read the information panel on the packaging for the exact amounts of fat and energy in processed foods. Do some comparison shopping – are those 'lite' items genuine in their implied promise? Whenever possible, choose fresh foods that you cook yourself rather than processed or packaged foods. This allows you to control the amount of fat that you are consuming at every meal.

Cue 7: Economy-size containers

Large container sizes prompt greater consumption. When a packet or container is large, many people have trouble monitoring the quantity of food they are consuming. This was illustrated in a study in which people were given stale, unfavourably tasting popcorn in different sized containers. Despite this unappetising fare, the subjects ate a whopping 49 per cent more when they were offered the popcorn in large buckets than they did when offered it in smaller ones.

Solution: Buy smaller containers and packages. If you prefer to buy the larger economy size of a product, repackage the food into portion-sized containers based on the label's serving size, especially if it is a snack food. Accordingly you will know how much you are eating. A superior alternative is to transfer the food from the container onto a plate.

Your daily bread

Many people ask me whether they should cut bread out of their diet altogether – because after all, bread is loaded with carbs and is fattening, right? But maybe wholegrain bread is okay? And white bread is the enemy? Not all breads are created equal. Let us slice through the misconceptions to find the healthiest of all.

Question: What are the health benefits of the different grains in multigrain bread?

Answer: Each whole grain possesses its own complement of phytochemicals (nutrients found in plants). In theory, the more grains, the more nutrients – and greater benefits. Certain multigrain breads contain mostly refined wheat flour and very little of the other grains. Even if they say seven-, nine- or twelve-grain, you should look for 'wholegrain' first on the ingredient list.

Question: Is white bread a nutritional zero?

Answer: Although the fibre, phytochemicals and trace minerals have all been refined out, white bread has some merit. Enriched with iron and B vitamins, including folic acid (which helps prevent birth defects), white bread is often fortified with calcium and is bulked up with cellulose (a form of fibre).

Question: Isn't wheat bread just white bread with a tan?

Answer: As with white bread, the phytochemicals and antioxidants have been refined out, but it is also enriched with the same nutrients as white bread. Although wheat bread contains about 25 per cent wholegrain flour, in terms of fibre content (it contains only about ½ to 1 gram per slice), it cannot compete with wholegrain bread.

Question: With sour dough, does heavy mean healthy?

Answer: Do not be fooled by the heft of sourdough – it comes from the starter used in the baking process, not from many, if any, whole grains. Although some specialty bakers do make wholegrain versions, most sourdoughs are no healthier than white or wheat breads.

Question: What about rye bread?

Answer: Much of the soft rye sold in supermarkets contains little whole grain. However, thin, dense loaves do contain it, as do some made by specialty bakers. Wholegrain rye contains lignans, which the body converts to enterolactone, an oestrogen-like molecule that may lower the risk of breast cancer. Look for caraway seeds on the ingredient list; these contain limonene and small amounts of perillyl alcohol, both potential cancer fighters.

Question: Pumpernickel is better for you because it is dark, right?

Answer: Not necessarily. The deep hue of most store-bought selections comes from molasses or caramel colouring, and most pumpernickels contain nothing more than refined wheat flour. True pumpernickel has a grainy texture, 1–2 grams of fibre per slice, and is made from wholegrain rye flour.

Question: Does raisin bread have any nutritional edge over white bread?

Answer: While raisins do contain potassium (which may lower blood pressure and the risk of stroke) and iron, most raisin breads are made with refined flour. A better choice would be one made with whole-wheat flour, which also contains nuts (a source of vitamin E and healthy monounsaturated fats).

Question: What is so good about whole-wheat bread?

Answer: For starters, phytic acid, a powerful antioxidant; flavonoids, other antioxidants; and oligosaccharides, indigestible compounds that may improve bowel health and immune function. This bread contains 2–4 grams of insoluble fibre per slice. Do not mistake regular wheat bread for whole-wheat; make sure the word 'whole-wheat' appears on the wrapper and at the top of the ingredient list.

SUMMING UP

* Always leave a little food on your plate – it demonstrates that you are in control.
* Be alert to cues that stimulate you to eat when you are not hungry.
* Develop strategies to deal with these cues and to simplify your life by: keeping food out of sight and out of reach; storing food in serving-size packages; cooking ample food to prevent excessive leftovers for second helpings and picking.
* Never eat until you are full.

SUCCESS STORY

Maria

I grew up as a chubby child and graduated into a fat adult. At 100 kilograms I stopped standing on the scales, because I was too embarrassed by the results. I was lazy and had a shocking diet. When I went travelling overseas I became a vegetarian, learned better food habits and started exercising. It wasn't so much becoming vegetarian that helped, it was not going for the easy food fixes such as McDonald's or KFC. While I was travelling I walked a lot more and started losing weight . . . and feeling better about myself.

I returned from overseas and continued to yo-yo between about 85 and 90 kilograms over the next few years. I gained the confidence to join a gym and watch my food habits, but I always was on some diet or another.

It's all about discipline. My downfall was having 'just one' of anything . . . I couldn't do it. One led to 10. I lacked willpower. People were continually commenting that I exercised more and ate better than most people. Things didn't add up and I was frustrated.

Arlene helped me find the discipline I needed. I learned to control the quantities of food – such as having a Freddo frog rather than a whole bar of chocolate, and having one glass of wine, not five. The other big change was to drop my gym membership, put on a pedometer and just walk . . . 10 000 steps every day.

My weight loss was steady, and within six months I reached a constant weight that I couldn't have even dreamed I'd be able to achieve: 67 kilograms. At close to 6 feet tall, I felt fantastic and healthy for the first time ever. It wasn't even that hard. I wished I'd started earlier!

Being vegetarian is a challenge in some respects, but the key is to control my intake of cheese, carbohydrates, smoothies and juices, and to be prepared with proper meat substitutes, such as legumes and tofu.

Comments from others that I looked like a model and was a leggy, thin brunette were welcome encouragement. However, some friends felt the change too radical and told me I looked sick and gaunt. They just wanted to retain the old me. In contrast, many comments like, 'Gee, the big-boned theory really isn't true' were very common and caused many to re-examine their own situation.

My true motivation was for my husband and me to start a family – I didn't want to start a pregnancy overweight and unhealthy. Well it worked. I am 16 weeks' pregnant and I feel wonderful. My daily walks continue, along with hopes of a bright future and the speedy return to a slim figure!

CHAPTER **9**

THE FIFTH COMMANDMENT:

Never feel deprived

This could seem a paradoxical commandment, given that I've just been telling you that you'll feel hungry as your body adjusts to smaller portion sizes. Feelings of deprivation – of being denied your favourite foods, or of being punished for being overweight by having to starve yourself – are the enemy of successful weight loss, and they only increase anxiety. Anxiety adds to stress and detracts from your sense of control, making it likely that sooner or later you'll binge on that 'forbidden' food.

It's human nature – if you feel that you can't have something you love, the 'want' is greater. It happened to me; I remember gorging on chocolate until I felt sick, in the hope I would never eat it again ... before I lapsed yet again!

I don't want you to go without. I don't want you to deny yourself anything you really love, as long as you plan for it and keep your portions small; the only thing you should deprive yourself of is *quantity*.

DON'T DENY YOURSELF

When people decide it's time to lose weight, they often mistakenly think there are entire categories of food that they are no longer allowed to eat, and this makes them miserable. For example, they assume they can never have dessert. That's absurd! You can't live your life without the piece of apple tart or chocolate cake that you really enjoy. Just have a little; you don't have to finish it. Cut a thin slice, put it on a plate, eat it slowly and enjoy every mouthful. My partner and I will order a dessert to share. We'll just have a few teaspoons and leave the rest. By having a taste we don't feel like we're missing out and it satisfies our craving.

If you're a chocoholic, like I used to be, you certainly don't have to go cold turkey. You can include lollies and chocolates in your eating plan; in fact, I suggest to some people that they have 30 grams – three squares – of chocolate every day. If you know that you can have a little treat every day, you feel satisfied and in control, whereas if you thought you weren't allowed any at all, you might binge on the whole bar. The trick is to savour every morsel – suck it, taste it and eat it slowly!

Knowing you can have something regularly will reduce your craving for it. My taste for chocolate has certainly diminished. I've gone from eating it all day with the regular binge, to the point now where I have a packet of chocolate biscuits in my cupboard that has been there for weeks.

Incorporate small quantities of anything you really enjoy into your eating plan. Men tend to prefer savoury foods, so it

Tiny treats

Question: My girlfriend and I go to the cinema every Saturday night and the candy bar is my downfall. I can't sit through a session without munching on something sweet, and I don't stop until I've finished the bag. Any suggestions?

Answer: Make it a smaller bag. Many candy bars, particularly those at the big multiplexes, allow you to help yourself from big containers and weigh individual lollies in a bag. If you buy a standard sealed bag containing twenty caramels or licorice allsorts, you're likely to eat every single one of them; but if you just put two or three into your bag, that's all you're going to eat. You don't have to miss out, provided you keep your portions small.

might be a burger and chips or a meat pie. It's perfectly possible to treat yourself to a burger once a week, if that's your fancy, provided your intake most of the time is balanced and sensible. Women generally prefer sweet things – chocolates, lollies, cakes and biscuits – in which case I'd suggest something like having a biscuit or a scone with jam twice a week for afternoon tea. However, remember that whatever you eat goes on a plate and you must sit down to enjoy it. Never eat out of the packet or standing up – you don't realise you are eating. If you really enjoy an alcoholic drink, it is possible to include that in your eating plan, but I urge caution – alcohol has no nutritional value and it also erodes your self-control (more on prudent alcohol consumption on page 164), often resulting in you eating more.

OUT OF SIGHT, OUT OF MIND

Occasionally enjoying your favourite foods doesn't mean that you should surround yourself with opportunities to indulge. Quite the contrary. Recognise your 'danger' foods, the ones that you find utterly irresistible. It might be cheese. Ice-cream. Crisps. Until you're convinced that you can control the quantities you will eat and won't be tempted to overindulge, don't keep them in the house. Eat them away from home where the portions are limited and access isn't so easy.

Janet, 39, personal assistant

Janet loves doughnuts. For years, she has had doughnuts for breakfast on her way to work, a ritual that was playing havoc with her waistline, but cutting them out altogether proved impossible. 'That's always been my downfall whenever I've tried to lose weight before,' she says. 'Because I saw them as off-limits, I craved them all the more.' This time Janet has organised her eating plan so that she can enjoy one of her favourite doughnuts with coffee for breakfast once a week. 'That's it – just once a week – yet somehow it seems to work for me. I really look forward to that doughnut every Tuesday morning and it helps me balance the rest of my intake for the week.'

Be wary of food you prepare ahead of time and keep close at hand, such as the packed lunch you take to work. Put it in the fridge or somewhere you can't see it until your lunch break, otherwise you'll eat it the minute you get peckish, and then have another lunch later. Keep low-fat nibbles such as carrot or cucumber sticks for those moments when temptation strikes.

Five holiday survival secrets

Holidays are times when we want to indulge ourselves. In fact, it can be hard not to, given that ice-cream is virtually synonymous with the seaside, and tempting meal deals are often included in holiday packages. Holidays are time out from real life, when our normal habits can fly out the window. How can you avoid overdoing it?

1. Don't make the mistake of crash-dieting to squeeze into a new swimsuit before you go away, or you will be so hungry when you arrive at your destination that you'll eat everything you feel you missed out on previously, and more! Rather, plan ahead and adopt healthy eating and exercise patterns months prior to your holiday, which will ensure you reach your desired weight and feel secure in your new lifestyle habits.

2. If you have booked an all-inclusive holiday that includes meals – particularly smorgasbords – remind yourself you don't have to eat everything because it is there. You

may have paid for as much as you can eat, but it's a poor bargain if you come home heavier than ever, and feeling uncomfortable too. Go once to the buffet table so you are aware of the quantity you are consuming.

3. Is everyone in the family having a ginormous ice-cream? If you really want one, skip lunch. Alternatively, why not just have a taste of theirs? A mouthful is often enough to satisfy your taste buds.

4. Watch the booze, which some people tend to overindulge on holiday; it relaxes your inhibitions and increases the likelihood you'll overdo your food intake.

5. Get physical. On holidays you have the time to walk or play sport that is so often lacking during your hectic workday schedule. Indulge in physical activity, not sweet treats or excess alcoholic beverages.

DON'T SKIP MEALS

The best way to avoid feeling deprived is to ensure you eat all your scheduled meals and snacks. This is essential, because allowing yourself to become famished can lead to disaster in the form of overeating and bingeing, often on the wrong food. Learn to listen to your body. What is your stomach telling you right now – that it's feeling satisfied, or maybe just a little peckish, or that it's ready to eat right now? Don't ignore the warning signs that you are becoming really hungry, and try not to miss a meal. If you do want to omit a meal, target dinner or supper.

While you will feel hungry for the first few weeks as your body adjusts to controlling the size of your portions, you are less likely to lose control if you know there is another meal soon. Your six daily meals and snacks add up to food every three hours; that's not too long to hold out. Don't keep yourself waiting. However busy you are, avoid the temptation to postpone eating until a more convenient moment, because you're likely to be ravenous when that moment finally arrives. Voracious hunger results in gobbling food and overeating, often on bad choices because that is the only food available.

KEEP IT REGULAR

Regular and predictable meal times – for example, breakfast at 7 a.m., lunch at 1 p.m., dinner at 7 p.m. and supper at 10 p.m. – help keep those hunger pangs under control. Try and stick to the same times each day. If, for example, you eat breakfast too early, you will push all your meals forward, which might sabotage your plans later in the evening.

So whatever you're doing, you *must* have breakfast, morning tea, lunch and afternoon tea. The only meal you could occasionally skip is dinner, because if you've had all your other meals throughout the day you might not be hungry by then and you're less likely to binge if you miss out now. If you have a big lunch, skip dinner or eat very little. Do not eat just because it is dinnertime. Two large meals result in too much food being consumed. Most of this eating is because we are accustomed to a large dinner and the availability of food. There is nothing stopping you from sitting with your family and chatting while they enjoy dinner, if you are not hungry.

Little changes add up to big losses

The trouble with the types of foods that most people relish is that they're not only loaded with fat and kilojoules, they're often very more-ish. How to ensure that you have just a little, not a lot, without feeling deprived? Try these tricks to fill up on your favourites while still slimming down.

Slice it right

Do you like pizza? How can you enjoy it without piling on the kilos? High-kilojoule extras such as sausage and pepperoni are a major no-no. Instead, pile on as many veggies as you like – they'll help fill you up. Ask your pizzeria to cut back on the cheese (some restaurants will use ricotta, which is an ideal alternative cheese).

Open your sandwich

Take the top off. By skipping that extra slice of bread, you save about 336 kilojoules per sandwich. Want an even lighter lunch? Try a Korean sandwich – beef and a light sauce wrapped in a lettuce leaf.

Transform your takeaway

When buying Chinese food, order some steamed or stir-fried vegetables along with your favourite chicken or prawn dish. Combine generous serves of the veggies with small portions of the other dishes in a bowl so you can see how much you are consuming. This way, you enjoy your favourite tastes with fewer kilojoules.

Pep up your pasta

There's nothing wrong with pasta or any other carbs such as bread or crackers. The problem is the portion size (and what you put on it, such as butter, cheese or creamy sauces). Some people eat enough for two in a single serving. You can still enjoy pasta, but why not bulk up your serving with vegetables tossed into a tomato-based sauce?

Downsize your snacks

Notice all those jumbo-sized bags of snacks – pretzels, baked potato chips and the like – that are available at the supermarket? They might seem tempting and economical if you're stocking up or have a big family, but they're also a pitfall for anyone wanting to lose weight. Never buy the big size of anything. Why? You will probably eat that whole big bag if it's in front of you. So pick up the snack-size packs instead. That way, you know exactly how much you are eating. I used to kid myself with the old 'I'll just have one handful' . . . until a few hours later I'd notice that three-quarters of the bag was gone. Of course, the bigger bag is often better value, so another way to downsize your snacks is to buy that large bag, but as soon as you get it home divide the snacks into small portions and store them in reusable containers. Keep them out of sight.

Dilute your drinks

One reason Australians have gained so much weight over the past twenty years is excessive liquid kilojoules. A few years ago there were no special coffees delivering up to 2100 kilojoules per serve. Coke came in a 200 ml bottle (equating to approximately 420 kilojoules), yet now we are confronted with 600 ml bottles: that's 1260 kilojoules, supposedly for one person! Cordials, soft drinks (including sports drinks) and even fruit juices are loaded with sugar, yet we swig them down to quench our thirst, unaware of just how high in energy they are. To limit all those liquid kilojoules, drink everything over ice or dilute beverages with tap or mineral water. Plain water, of course, is the best thirst-quencher and it is kilojoule-free, and fortified with fluoride, which is good for your teeth.

THE LOWDOWN ON POPULAR DIETS

People associate diets with deprivation, and fad diets are based on this idea. If, for example, you're on a high-protein diet, you are depriving yourself of carbohydrates; this is not normal eating. Weird and wonderful diets grab your attention and keep your motivation up ... for a while. However, they are usually quite difficult to maintain over the long haul.

There is an abundance of dietary advice in the weight-loss section of the bookshop. How do you distinguish the duds/fad diets from the diets that offer sound nutritional advice? Let us take a closer look at several popular offerings and sort the good (most have a few useful suggestions) from the bad (fad diets that won't last the distance).

The Atkins Diet

Let us begin with the most controversial diet of them all – the high-protein, low-carb Atkins diet.

What's good: Following Atkins *will* make the scale go down. A study published in the *New England Journal of Medicine* showed that people following Atkins for six months lost 7 kilograms compared with a loss of 3 kilograms by those following a classic low-fat, high-carbohydrate plan. Plus you get to eat meat, cheese, eggs and butter – paradise for protein lovers!

What's bad: That same study found that after a year there was no significant difference in weight loss between the Atkins group and the classic dieters. Atkins advocates eating many foods high in saturated fat and avoiding certain vegetables and fruits – a risky approach, since unprocessed produce is packed with vitamins, minerals, fibre and water; all essential to good health as well as sustainable weight loss. The jury is still out on the long-term health implications of this program. However, while it is in vogue to be anti-carbohydrate, scientists agree that successful weight loss is not about carbs, it is about kilojoules. Expending more kilojoules in physical activity than you are consuming is the key to successful slimming.

The bottom line: In the initial stages of this diet you eliminate almost all carbs, which does make your weight go down – but you are losing water as well as fat. Because food choices are limited, fewer kilojoules are consumed – the key to any weight-loss plan. If you do decide to go on the Atkins Diet, most weight-loss experts (myself included) advise only following it short term. If you want to try it for a few weeks as a jump-start, fine. After that, you are better off opting for moderate amounts of lean protein and pairing it with sensible portions of salads, vegetables, fruit and whole grains, because these contain the fibre, vitamins and minerals your body requires.

The GI Revolution

This is one of a series of books focusing on the benefits of consuming foods with a low glycaemic index (GI). Originally targeting people with diabetes, this regime has become very popular for weight loss.

What's good: The lower the GI of the food you're consuming, the higher its satiety and the longer before you start feeling hungry again. Low-GI foods boost blood sugar more slowly; these generally include high-fibre foods such as whole grains, legumes, as well as low-carbohydrate foods such as meats. Most fruits and vegetables have a relatively low GI ranking because of their fibre content.

What's bad: A problem with using GI is that it is based on consuming food in isolation. For example, if you eat a high-GI food such as white bread and combine it with a low-GI food such as peanut butter, the peanut butter will balance the meal's 'glycaemic load'. In addition, GI is no indication of how healthy the food is. Ice-cream, which contains a mix of saturated fat and sugar, has a surprisingly low GI, whereas a banana, which is loaded with potassium and is very healthy, has a high GI. Exercise will also affect your glycaemic response. If you exercise regularly, glucose is cleared from your bloodstream more quickly, no matter what you eat. In addition, if you add fat or protein to a meal and eat it slowly, a lower glycaemic response will result.

The bottom line: It is somewhat obsessive – you can have this rice but not that rice, this potato but not that potato – and focusing on low GI can still result in an unhealthy diet. I believe in eating everything in moderation, making wise choices of high fibre and fewer processed foods while still allowing 'treats' in small portions.

The Body Shaping Diet

This advocates that women tailor their eating plan to their particular body type:

- gynoid (bottom heavy)
- android (top heavy)
- thyroid (lean with fine-boned limbs and a slender neck)
- lymphatic (round-shaped with thick, straight limbs).
  The type of food you eat depends on your body type.

What's good: Nothing much.

What's bad: The premise is absurd. In reality, there is not much difference between the dietary recommendations for the different body shapes.

The bottom line: You were born with the genes that determine your figure type, which cannot be altered by eating particular foods. While you can reduce the total amount of fat on your body, you certainly can't alter its basic shape (apart from resorting to plastic surgery).

Eat Right for Your Type

This oddly named fad has its fair share of believers, despite having no scientific basis to back it up. The theory goes like this: If you and your best friend are the same height and the same age, but she has blood type A and you have type B, then you should follow different eating regimes.

What's good: This diet requires you to identify your blood type, which is valuable health information.

What's bad: Its main argument – that it is your blood type that determines the type of foods you should consume, not your total kilojoule intake that causes you to gain weight.

The bottom line: I do not know of any doctor or dietary authority that endorses this idea, nor have I seen any study that backs it up. Restricting your kilojoule intake and increasing your activity level will assist weight loss, but this has nothing to do with your blood type. My advice: give it a miss.

The Liver Cleansing Diet

A worldwide bestseller a few years back, this diet is still popular.

What's good: It's a low-fat eating plan, which will reduce your cholesterol level along with your weight. It also promotes exercise as part of the plan.

What's bad: It incorporates faddish elements; for example, it advocates cutting out items like chocolate and cake altogether. Normal eating doesn't require removing certain foods completely; it allows having them in small portions occasionally. This diet also advocates the use of various vitamins and minerals, which, if you eat normally, you should not require. The rationale – that weight gain is due to a sluggish or toxic liver – is dubious; you don't need to detox if you're living a healthy lifestyle.

The bottom line: You will lose weight on this diet, which is a healthy eating plan, although it is somewhat restrictive, which could make it difficult to adhere to long term.

The Zone
The favoured diet in Hollywood a while ago, and still going strong.

What's good: The plan is easy to follow and encourages you to reduce your food intake by reducing portion sizes.

What's bad: It is just an 1100-calorie (4620-kilojoule) diet in disguise, which most dieticians say is too stringent over the long haul. Plus, the Zone claims that dividing your daily intake of kilojoules into 40 per cent carbs, 30 per cent protein and 30 per cent fat will help you attain a metabolic state that will keep you thin. I don't think so! Eating small meals throughout the day certainly keeps your metabolism ticking over nicely, but this has nothing to do with the Zone's 40/30/30 percentages.

The bottom line: Short term, the Zone works. The program – and related products sold with it – is simply a gimmick to get you to eat less. If the 40/30/30 rule helps take the guesswork out of dieting, go for it. Just don't fall for its pseudo-science.

Sugar Busters

What started as a fringe diet went mainstream a few years back with a bestselling book.

What's good: Some information could help diabetics.

What's bad: This plan urges you to eliminate or drastically reduce foods with a high GI (foods that quickly convert to sugar in the body, leading to an insulin spike followed by a crash). This advice may be useful to diabetics but is less relevant to most other people. For example, the original Sugar Busters book defined carrots – a high-GI food – as a no-no. Think about that for a moment: Are the carrots you like to snack on *really* the reason you have gained weight?

The bottom line: Sugar is not the problem. This diet claims that sugar causes diabetes and is a risk factor for heart disease, and that insulin causes weight gain – none of this is true. Additionally, the dietary advice is inconsistent: it recommends limiting your intake of saturated fat, but its list of acceptable foods includes cream, butter, cheese, milk, pork and 'lean' beef. It also restricts or excludes healthy foods such as carrots, corn, beetroot and bananas, and it is also low in calcium. You have been warned!

The South Beach Diet

The hottest fad on the market, it is sold out in many bookstores.

What's good: As with the Atkins Diet, you're given permission to indulge your cravings for meat, cheese, bacon and eggs.

What's bad: In the first two-week phase, you must eliminate bread, potatoes, pasta, baked goods, lollies, biscuits, ice-cream, sugar and alcohol. Few slimmers succeed by going cold turkey on their favourite foods.

The bottom line: The South Beach Diet claims you will drop 4–6 kilograms in the first phase. Sounds great but think about it. To shed just half a kilo, you must expend 14 700 more kilojoules than you consume. To lose the promised 6 kilograms requires the expenditure of 191 100 kilojoules over a fortnight. That would require burning 13 650 kilojoules a day – the equivalent of running a marathon – for two weeks straight, which is scarcely realistic.

Which brings me to a point that most fad diets skim over – the importance of exercise in any weight-loss routine. Few programs mention the fact that when you restrict your eating, your metabolism starts to slow down. The only way to reverse this trend is to commence strength-building and aerobic exercise. More on this topic in Chapter 13.

SUMMING UP

* Don't cut out your favourite treats completely, you'll only crave them more. Just have a little, not a lot. The only thing I want you to deprive yourself of is quantity.
* Don't surround yourself with temptation; keep foods you're likely to binge on out of sight.
* Never let yourself get too hungry or you'll binge. Be sure to eat all your meals and snacks.
* If you do drop a meal because you're not hungry, make it dinner, not breakfast or lunch.

SUCCESS *Peter* STORY

As far as weight control is concerned, I have been through it all. I have been overweight for most of my life. I grew up in a family hotel, with buffet breakfasts and lunches and *table d'hôte* dinners. My favourite, of course, were those Sunday buffets, where there was unlimited tucker and scrumptious cream desserts that I could never resist.

Soon after leaving the hotel, I went on one of the many milkshake diets. I lost 10 kilograms in five months, but as soon as I started eating a normal diet again, the weight poured back on – within weeks. Not only did I regain the weight lost, but some more to boot.

I tried visiting a dietician, slimming vitamins, prescribed weight management tablets, weight clubs, the tomato soup diet (and the like), and lost the same

10 kilograms regularly, gaining a few kilograms each unsuccessful time.

I eventually gave up on my weight-loss efforts and took the line of least resistance: I bought new, bigger clothes, because my old ones all seemed to have shrunk in the washing machine and the new cuts were so skimpy!

After my son was born my doctor suggested that my son would soon be visiting me in the cardiac ward if I did not reduce my weight. He told me of a dietician who was hard but got results. This tactic seemed to press the right buttons – I realised I had a responsibility to my wife and son to sort out my health problems.

Arlene has given me a liveable lifestyle. Instead of having a takeaway Thai pasta lunch at my desk, I began visiting the gym for 20 minutes. Eventually I cancelled my gym membership and walked for the full lunch hour, instead of spending half the time waiting for a locker, waiting for a treadmill, waiting for the shower. I would then grab a salad, sandwich or some fresh sushi to eat after my walk each day. After a while, the lunchtime walk wasn't challenging enough, so I started to walk the 7 kilometres home.

As the kilograms came off, the more I got motivated and the easier it was to stick to my lifestyle plan. Unfortunately, however, temptation could not always be avoided. At these weight-gain times it would have been so easy to 'go off the rails' and revert to my old bad habits. Arlene helped me get back on track. She was always supportive but demanding and advised how I could best cope with the situation.

My doctor initially suggested that I lose 10 per cent of my body weight – I am now down more than 20 per cent and I feel wonderful. Even my blood results think I am a different person. In less than a year, my weight loss was equivalent to 50 × 500 g tubs of butter and still counting. The aches and pains have disappeared, and the weight has gone, forever.

CHAPTER 10

THE SIXTH COMMANDMENT:

Make a meal of it

Food is one of life's great pleasures, but it must be given the attention and respect it deserves. Do not graze and snack all day, guzzle junk food straight from the packet or nibble food directly from the fridge. Sit down to eat, relax and enjoy your meal, instead of rushing and devouring food as you are walking down the street. Food is not just fuel, something to be shovelled down as fast as possible before continuing with the next activity. This kind of consumption invariably results in you overeating without even savouring the food – what a pity you haven't taken the time to take pleasure in the meal. In addition, the extra kilojoules you are unaware of consuming are causing you to gain weight.

You are not even enjoying the food! Most of the time you are scarcely aware that you have eaten, because you are not focusing your attention on the food. This is mindless eating, and mindless eating piles on the kilos. If you don't know or care what you are putting in your mouth, you are not in control of your eating . . . and that, as we have seen, will not help you reach and maintain a healthy weight.

Remember the days when the family would congregate at the end of the day to share the evening meal and discuss the day's events? I recall how when I was a child my family used to sit around the dinner table and chat about what had happened during the day. Those times are unfortunately gone. Few families today ever sit down to dinner together. Dinner? This one is coming home late because he is at soccer, that one is coming home even later because she is at work and the little ones have probably eaten early in front of the television (a very bad habit, see box on page 156 for more). Breakfast? Eaten on the run – a muesli bar on the bus – if it is eaten at all. Some families do not have set mealtimes – everyone just grabs something from the fridge and heads off to work, school or a social event.

Why do we choose to live this way? Our lives are pressured and rushed. We are often tired and stressed, and we are not enjoying our meals in a relaxed and leisurely fashion. We are not thinking about what we are eating, we are just gobbling 'easy' meals. This is not just nutritionally bad, it also impacts family life because we are missing out on the daily contact.

NEVER EAT STANDING

Always sit down at a table to eat, even if you are only having a snack. Never eat standing up; if you sit down you will focus more on your food and are more likely to notice what – and how much – you are eating. Yet almost everywhere you look in the street you can see people walking around with ice-creams or packets of chips. Typically these people do not see such items as 'food', so they are oblivious to the kilojoules that they are consuming as they rush about their business. It's easy to munch through copious kilojoules in the kitchen while preparing meals, serving the family or tidying up; I have to exercise self-control to not pick while I clear the table. If, however, you stop and sit down every time you eat, you are actually aware of what you put into your mouth.

PUT IT ON A PLATE

Always put food on a plate before you commence eating. Many people stand in the kitchen and eat out of the fridge. Consider the average workplace: there is a biscuit jar in the tearoom, and when staff members pass the jar they invariably grab a biscuit. They are seldom aware of what they are doing, so they probably consume many more biscuits than they realise. It is much better to take that biscuit, put it on a plate and sit down and enjoy it with a cup of tea or coffee or a glass of water.

Putting your food on a plate makes you aware of exactly how much and what you are eating, and it enables you to control your portion size. It also makes a ritual of mealtimes, allowing you to relax and enjoy your food rather than mindlessly picking.

Ideally, you will do this at each meal. However, life is not always ideal, so you must always try your best depending on the situation. Sophie, a busy social worker, has so many appointments that she often cannot leave the office for an appropriate lunch break. She does, however, make the effort to sit down at her desk to eat her lunch, shutting her door with the intention that she is not interrupted. Accordingly, she is able to give her full attention to her food, enjoy it, and have a few moments of relaxation.

TREAT YOURSELF

If you were entertaining guests, you would not give them a hot dog in a serviette or on a paper plate, would you? You would put a fresh cloth on the table, lay it with your best

Keep track of the snacks

Question: I eat very little and still cannot lose weight. What is going wrong?

Answer: You are probably consuming more food than you think, and not necessarily at mealtimes. Frequent unconscious snacks can add up to a lot of energy over the day, without you realising it. Try keeping a diary of every single thing you put in your mouth — including all leftovers, nibbles and tastes, to that handful of peanuts or square of chocolate. Ensure all your food is put on a plate and you are sitting down, and that you do not eat on the run or standing up. You will be astonished to discover the number of extra kilojoules you have been consuming!

crystal, china and cutlery, and put out a vase of flowers. You might light candles, and you would put appropriate serviettes on the table. A special meal would be prepared. All this effort is to ensure that your guests have a wonderful time.

Well, if that is the manner in which you treat your friends, are you not worthy of the same effort? Why not make every meal special, whether you are eating with friends, family or alone? It does not have to be formal; it should just have some sense of occasion – to serve even a snack on a nice plate, to drink plain water from an elegant glass. It might take a few seconds longer, but it does not cost any more to serve yourself with style. It does have surprising psychological benefits.

It is often said that food is an expression of love, and how we present it certainly says a lot about our feelings towards the person on the receiving end. When that person is you, it does nothing for your self-esteem – or your waistline – when the message being sent is that you are not worth worrying about. This is particularly pertinent if you are single or eating alone. It is easy to adopt bad habits, because you simply cannot be bothered looking after number one – yourself!

There are other reasons apart from your self-esteem and good nutrition to make an occasion of every meal and snack. If you are eating smaller portions than you are accustomed to, you are less likely to feel deprived if you put the food on a plate, make it look attractive (a sprig of parsley) and give it your undivided attention. You will probably enjoy it more because you have given yourself the time to notice what you are eating. Simply putting something on a plate and sitting

Russell's story

Russell, a journalist, works long hours meeting demanding deadlines and often does not return home until ten or eleven at night. By then he is usually ravenous as well as exhausted. Instead of preparing a balanced dinner, he consumes anything he can find in the kitchen. Russell knew that this was not a healthy or pleasurable way of eating, so he decided that he would change his habits and start taking a prepared meal to work. He now heats the food in the microwave during a break around 7 p.m., and sits down in the staffroom to enjoy his dinner. Russell is more productive at work now that he is not frenetically hungry, and when he gets home late, already having consumed his evening meal, he goes straight to bed.

down to eat slows you down, which translates into you being more satisfied, sooner, with less food.

There are also clear cues when the meal begins and ends – it begins with putting food on the plate and sitting down to eat it, and it ends when you have finished and cleared the dishes from the table. This is completely different from snatching food on the run – without such cues, you are less likely to feel that you have actually eaten a meal, so you are more likely to eat much more over the course of a day than if you had simply sat down for each meal.

The French approach to food is to view a mealtime as an opportunity to socialise as well as enjoy a meal. Why not try

How television makes you fat

Don't eat in front of the television. When your attention is distracted from your food intake, your enjoyment of your meal will decrease and the volume you consume will increase. A particular problem can arise: you begin to associate eating with watching television, so simply switching on becomes a subconscious trigger to eat. The advertisements for fatty, high-kilojoule foods – pizzas, hamburgers, chocolates and the like; seldom fruit or vegetables – give you extra stimulus to eat more. So, watch television before or after, but never during a meal. Organise other activities, such as knitting, to keep your hands busy while you are watching television.

it? Make a daily date with your family to get together over dinner at a certain time. Avoid creating a rushed or confronting atmosphere; make mealtimes relaxed occasions during which you talk over the day's events.

Vary the mix

There are more ways to eat in style than simply setting an elegant table. Start by being a little adventurous with your food choices. You would not watch the same episode of your favourite television show week after week. Yet when it comes to diet, many of us are stuck on re-run meals, consuming the same familiar items virtually every day. It is a habit – we feel safe with what we are accustomed to – but we would benefit from being more adventurous. Lack of variety can deprive you of valuable nutrients, and it can also result in food cravings, bingeing and weight gain. Restricted food choices become increasingly less satisfying, which could prompt you to impulse-eat, make incorrect food choices or increase your portion sizes.

Make changes. Vary your menus regularly. Try to include as many different items in your daily intake as possible (soups, salads, stir-fries and other dishes that include lots of different ingredients). Sample the cuisine of other cultures, and spice up your meals with new tastes and flavours (more on this topic in Chapter 12).

SUMMING UP

* Do not eat standing or walking – always sit down.
* Never eat food from a packet or from the fridge. Put the food on a plate.
* Serve yourself the same way as you would a guest.
* Avoid distractions such as television while eating.
* Make every meal an occasion so that you are aware that you have eaten and will feel more satisfied.

SUCCESS STORY
Antoinette

I have been overweight for as long as I can remember, even though I would classify myself as the 'sporty' type. Hurtful taunts about my weight were a part of my younger years, and I felt very insecure about myself and my friendships. When I joined the workforce and had my own income, I made a lot of bad food choices and my weight escalated. Two pregnancies really compounded my weight problems.

The years and the weight rolled on until I took the extreme step and had my stomach stapled. I lost nearly 30 kilograms, but without the help of a dietician I eventually reverted back to my mildly bad eating habits until I eventually regained the 30 kilograms. Recently I realised the years were passing, as were my dreams of trekking holidays in both Australia and overseas. By this stage I had so many niggling physical problems that I decided I had to do something NOW.

My physiotherapist put me in touch with a woman who taught Pilates, so I signed up for classes. Although I was not losing any weight, a lot of my aches and pains were disappearing. When I began working with Arlene and the weight slowly came off, she encouraged me and I gained enough confidence to join a gym. As I started to get a few compliments on my weight loss, my attitude became more positive and I settled into a regular exercise routine, which involved a variety of training over six days of the week, with Sunday being a rest day for my body.

I am now beginning to see the light at the end of the tunnel. To think it all started with Arlene insisting on my walking 10 000 steps every day!

CHAPTER 11

THE SEVENTH COMMANDMENT:

Eat slowly

Eating slowly helps you control your intake. It takes 20 minutes from the time you begin eating to the time your brain receives the message from your stomach that food has been consumed. During those 20 minutes, if you eat quickly it is possible to devour an abundance of food – much more than you need, and more than you would eat if you registered that your appetite had been satisfied.

MORE TIME = FEWER KILOJOULES

Remember the French approach to food described in Chapter 7? An interesting difference between the eating styles of the French and the Australians was the fact that the French do not just eat smaller portions than we do, but they take longer to eat them. The average French person devotes nearly 100 minutes a day to eating, while Australians swallow their daily bread in only 60 minutes. The French take longer to eat less, which could be one of the reasons why only 10 per cent of them are obese versus 30 per cent of Australians.

> *'Festina lente (hasten slowly)'*
>
> ⬩
>
> LATIN PROVERB

Paradoxically, the more time you take to eat, the fewer kilojoules you consume ... and the more likely you are to enjoy your food, because you are able to give it the attention and respect it requires.

Slow eating will allow you to take the utmost pleasure in your meal. I went to an obesity presentation where the lecturer gave us all a single delicious chocolate to eat. He would not permit us to chew and swallow it; he made us taste it, suck it and really take our time savouring every morsel. When we had finished it we felt that one square was adequate. Had we eaten it as quickly as people normally gulp down chocolate, we would have devoured more in the same time, but not appreciated and enjoyed it as much. Solution? Relish every morsel of food and eat it slowly, and you will find that you no longer need or want large quantities.

SAVOUR THE FLAVOUR

It is impossible to enjoy your meal if you devour it rapidly. We have become accustomed to living in the fast lane. We rush from one thing to another – work, social commitments, picking up the kids, shopping – and this includes hurrying through our meals. Gobbling has become a bad habit.

Industries are encouraging us to eat quickly and on the run, which means eating more; this translates into bigger profits for fast-food operators. A lot of 'junk' food requires very little chewing. There is not much to chew in fast-food hamburgers, pizzas, ice-cream, milkshakes and the like, so you can gulp down a lot very quickly, without realising the quantity you are consuming. Try eating a salad before a meal – you have to chew it thoroughly, which slows the eating process.

Little losses add up

You do not have to pig out to put on weight. A very little overindulgence results in weight gain over time. For example, just an extra 210 kilojoules excess intake each day will result in a gain of up to 1 kilogram per year; over several years, this can add a lot to your waistline. However, you might not have to deny yourself too much to lose it again. If you forgo that extra 210 kilojoules a day you will maintain your weight at a stable level, and if you eat 420 fewer kilojoules per day you will actually start to lose weight. That equates to a slice of bread a day – not too much of a sacrifice!

BEAT THE BLOAT

Many people only stop eating when they feel full or bloated. I remember before I took control of my eating I used to undo my zip after dinner because I was so overfed! Many of us equate satiety (the feeling of having had enough to eat) with feeling quite stuffed, and it can take some time to adjust to eating only until you are comfortable, not full. Often overweight people complain of bloating, flatulence and reflux (heartburn). This is because the volume of food they are consuming is too large and is pushing everything up and out. Eating too quickly only exacerbates the problem. The solution? Slow down, and eat less.

GO SLOW

If you have always eaten rapidly, it will take a conscious effort to eat slowly. Here are some tips to get you started.

- Have a (non-alcoholic) drink before starting on the food; this will slow you down, and at the same time it will fill you with fluid. Water – plain or sparkling – is ideal, but tea or even a cappuccino does the trick in the colder months. Take pleasure in the drink while everybody is busy with the bread basket. It will take the edge off your hunger, so you can relax and enjoy your meal.

- Start with a first course that takes time to eat. A salad containing lettuce, rocket, cucumber, capsicum, onion and carrot needs lots of chewing. Hot soup is a good option because you cannot consume it quickly; try a chewy variety such as bean or chunky vegetable. When you have finished, you will feel satisfied and able to take your time with the next course – or maybe not even bother with it at all.

- Cut a small piece of food, put it in your mouth and then put the knife and fork down. Chew it well. Do not pick your knife and fork up until you have swallowed the mouthful. Now cut another small piece, and go through the process again.

- Focus on your food and make a conscious effort to

register the taste of everything you put in your mouth.
- You cannot eat and talk at the same time, so involve yourself in the conversation at the dinner table. Chatting with friends and family over a meal transforms it from a fuel stop to a pleasant social occasion. Aim to be the last to finish, not the first.
- Take five. Simply slowing down – just by taking a 5-minute pause between courses, or even in the middle of a single course – offers your body a chance to say 'Hey, enough!'

Luke's story

Luke is a corporate lawyer who is always on the go. He regularly puts in 16-hour days, often flying interstate to see clients and grabbing meals along the way. Luke usually ate with his mobile phone beside his plate, taking several calls during each meal. 'I realised that I was trying to beat not just the clock, but the phone, because I was eating faster and faster to finish before it rang again,' he recalls. Luke often suffered indigestion, bloating and reflux. He felt stressed continuously. Finally he realised he had to make some changes. His first step was an obvious solution: he turned off the phone during meals. His indigestion improved. The next step Luke took was to schedule a break for lunch and dinner, in which he did nothing but eat . . . slowly . . . and enjoy his meal. He is now on his way towards normalising his eating – and his life. He has time to relax and catch his breath in an otherwise hectic schedule.

Booze control

Go slow on alcohol. With more than 420 kilojoules in a single shot, alcoholic drinks can add kilos fast. Here are some tips on how to make smart beverage choices.

Eat before you drink

Drinking on an empty stomach speeds alcohol absorption into your bloodstream. Drinking while you are hungry can also encourage overindulgence in salty, fatty bar snacks such as nuts and crisps; these only increase your thirst and encourage you to drink more alcohol. If you have a proper meal before you go out for a drink, you are more likely to stay on track . . . and in charge.

Drink before you drink

If you are thirsty, you will gulp down alcoholic beverages in greater quantities than you planned. Have plenty of water before that big night out.

Space out the alcohol

Alcohol dehydrates you, so drink plenty of water throughout the evening. Alternate every alcoholic drink with a non-alcoholic drink.

Dilute your drinks

Cut down the alcohol in alcoholic drinks with low-kilojoule mixers, such as diet cola or diet tonic water, or make a spritzer by topping up your white wine with soda water. A glass of white wine filled with ice is very refreshing!

Stick to your limit

Resolve to have just one drink, two at most, and then switch to non-alcoholic drinks. Beware of waiters or hosts intent on refilling your glass, because this makes it hard to keep track.

Fake it

If friends are pressuring you to drink more than you intended to – in a 'shout' situation, for example – and you fear being seen as a party pooper if you refuse, why not fake it? Order yourself a non-alcoholic drink that looks like the real thing. Who can tell the difference between a gin and tonic and a sparkling water on the rocks with a twist of lime and a swizzle stick?

Nix the 'nog

Eggs, milk, sugar, brandy . . . eggnog isn't a drink, it's a dessert, with over 840 kilojoules in a 150 gram serving! So give it a miss, and also watch out for kilojoule-laden cocktails.

WATER WORKS

How many people have told you that drinking lots of water – at least eight glasses a day – will help you lose weight? Drinking water in itself does not cause you to lose weight. However, water will definitely fill your stomach and consequently you will feel less hungry and might eat less. Your body doesn't treat water as food so it won't have any long-term effect on your appetite. It is a good idea to stay well hydrated, both for general health and so you do not mistake thirst for hunger, and overeat. I do not believe in forcing yourself to drink too much water. The fluid your body needs is present in numerous sources – including fruit, vegetables, tea and other beverages, soup and jelly – which should be included in a healthy, balanced diet.

SUMMING UP

* Take your time at the table – you will enjoy your meals more and feel satisfied with less food.
* Stop eating as soon as you feel comfortable – do not con-tinue until you feel full.

SUCCESS STORY

Ben

As a child and through most of my life I did not have a problem with my weight. Even into my forties there was not a real problem. I started gaining weight slowly over the latter years, and even though my doctor made regular comments (because I suffered from high blood pressure), I put it down to age – middle-age spread, body shape changing as one gets older, and lifestyle. I didn't eat unhealthy food, I just had too much of a good thing.

My doctor told me that unless I lost weight – apart from my high blood pressure – I would have to go onto medication for diabetes. I was not self-motivated enough to lose the weight, so she recommended I seek help from a dietician.

Over the past five months with Arlene's motivation and help I have learned to eat little and often, and everything in moderation. I have also learned the importance of exercise, in my case an hour and a half of brisk walking daily. In the past five months I have lost 18 kilograms. I feel healthier, I have more energy, and my last blood test results showed lowered blood pressure (the best in years), normal cholesterol and no trace of diabetes.

I have had no problems following this regime. I don't feel deprived. With a certain amount of discipline I intend to sit on my ideal weight of 90 kilograms. People have been very generous with their praise and compliments, saying I look ten years younger!

CHAPTER 12

THE EIGHTH COMMANDMENT:

Enjoy your food

Food is an essential part of life. It nourishes you, fuels your activities and is the basis of many social gatherings. You must never feel guilty about the food you are enjoying – meals are a time to be self-indulgent. I want you to savour every morsel you consume. After all, food is one of the primary joys of life!

Nutritious food must taste good. Never waste a meal – each one must be delicious and prepared to your liking. Not every meal is memorable, and many may be repetitious, but you should make an effort to incorporate the variety your tastebuds demand into your meals.

Our hurried lifestyle affects our eating behaviour. When you are rushed and disorganised you will often have to be content to eat processed food, fast food or food out of packets or boxes. These dishes are seldom out of choice, but the disordered situation demands an easy solution for a meal when you are hungry and tired. These foods are generally high in salt and fat, and low in fibre – not the most nutritious selection. In addition, generally they will not satisfy all your senses or nourish your body. They are generally eaten on the run – you are often not aware you have had a meal!

Never miss out on the sweetness or smell of a ripe mango, the tangy taste of lemon juice or the silky texture of a fresh oyster, with its brinish aftertaste. Savour the warmth of a thick barley soup or a hearty·casserole on a cold winter's night. The flavours and smells stimulate all your senses and lift your spirits while supplying your body with the nutrients it requires.

The colours, textures and aromas enhance the eating experience. Imagine the irresistible smell of hot bread, roasting meat or piping-hot vegetable soup – makes your mouth water, doesn't it? The crunch of capsicum, carrots, cucumber and other vegetables bring a salad to life. Think of the attraction of a fresh fruit salad with its bright and varied colours.

The sound of food cooking – sizzling beef at a Chinese restaurant as they bring the griddle to the table, popcorn popping – creates an exciting sensation. The soft pop when you bite into a perfect grape or the satisfying snap of a snow pea between your teeth. Food is a feast for all the senses, not only the tastebuds.

Hunger increases your enjoyment of a meal; smelling the food, tasting the food and stimulating every sensory organ increases your satiety. When you have quality, you don't need quantity to feel satisfied, so whatever you eat must be the best! You must be hungry when you eat, you must relish every morsel. Now that you are consuming smaller portions, they must be as delicious as possible. Controlling your intake of energy is no excuse for removing flavour and variety. The tastier the meal, the more satisfied you will be with less.

> *'Variety is the spice of life'*

You must not deny your taste-buds. Eat slowly, to give yourself the time to savour each mouthful and the various flavours. You should not have to reach for the saltshaker (too much salt can ruin the natural flavour and harm your health); rather, utilise the myriad spices, herbs and condiments that turn insipid into irresistible.

INCREASING MEAL APPEAL

Impress your family and yourself with meal preparation and presentation. Attractive food tastes better. It's so easy to turn a plain meal into a flavoursome feast. Try these ideas.

- Marinate meat in lemon juice, wine and vinegar.
- Season foods with fresh and dried herbs or condiments – dill with fish, mint with lamb, cranberry sauce with turkey, mustard on beef, lemon grass with Asian dishes. Use parsley, sage, rosemary, thyme, garlic, marjoram, oregano and bay leaves, which add taste and relish to so many savoury dishes, from soups to casseroles.
- Sauce up your meals with Worcestershire, barbecue, sweet chilli, soy or black bean sauces.
- Some like it hot – use horseradish, pepper, chilli, mustard and curry pastes (not satay) and powders.

- Add interest to fruit and sweet dishes with cinnamon, all-spice, nutmeg and vanilla. Ginger adds tang to sweet and savoury dishes alike.
- Eat your food freshly cooked and increase its eye appeal with attractive garnishes, smart plating and other touches you see in magazines, cookbooks and restaurants.
- Become adventurous and try different recipes, foods from a variety of ethnic groups, fruits and vegetables. The numerous cuisines and ingredients available in Australia could add to the excitement of your meal repertoire and prevent boredom.

Are you eating your feelings?

Why do some people bury their sorrows in a tub of ice-cream, while others crunch their way through a bag of chips? After years of observing how people use food to deal with negative emotions, I put it down to what I call head hunger and heart hunger. I believe that feelings of stress, frustration, irritation or self-disgust (emotions stemming from head hunger) or empty feelings such as boredom, depression or loneliness (heart hunger) make people crave foods with particular physical properties. These include chewy foods (caramels, muesli bars, sultanas), crunchy foods (nuts, crackers, cereal), textured items (French fries, hot dogs, pizza), soft, creamy food (ice-cream, chocolate, cheese), 'comfort' food (puddings, cakes, biscuits) and childhood favourites (casseroles, homemade bread, Mum's cooking).

It is essential to distinguish head and heart hunger from stomach hunger, which is when you genuinely need food. You must always have a snack or meal when you are 'stomach hungry', or you will trigger the urge to binge. When your cravings relate to head or heart hunger, consider other methods to release stress and indulge yourself without turning to food (exercise is ideal).

Brian's story

Brian gained weight when his marriage ended. His wife had always been responsible for the grocery shopping and cooking. Brian's cooking skills were limited. He didn't know how to prepare salads, shop for fruit and vegetables, or keep easy consumables like yoghurt, cottage cheese or canned tuna. His limit was grills, barbecues, takeaways and fried foods – endless steaks, eggs, sausages, bacon, chops, chips and schnitzels that were quick and easy. The meals soon became boring. The food was unbalanced and high in fat, and Brian found himself overeating to assuage his desire for a delicious meal. A friend in a similar situation suggested a solution: 'Around the world in seven days'. They would attempt a recipe from a different cuisine every night of the week. Brian took up the challenge. He tried Indian, Mexican, Thai, Italian, Lebanese, Chinese and an Aussie burger. Brian realised that cooking could be fun and that he was able to create appetising meals. He started buying cookbooks filled with ideas to use spices, condiments and herbs – his meals were now healthy, exciting and delicious.

CRANK UP THE FLAVOUR – NOT THE FAT, SALT OR SUGAR

Fat adds flavour. It is true. Fast food and processed food manufacturers bump up the fat, salt and sugar in their products – it is a cheap and easy way to make them tasty and filling. Steamed vegetables do get boring!

Fat

You should not eliminate fat completely. Fat in small quantities is essential for your body to absorb certain vitamins – however, in excess it will rapidly escalate your kilojoule intake. Fat in processed foods is generally unhealthy saturated or trans fat. Remember that gram for gram, fat contains almost twice the kilojoule content of carbohydrates and proteins, so treat yourself to small portions of only the very best products. Enjoy your small portion of chocolate, cake, or ice-cream. Be aware of what you are consuming, and savour every morsel. Attempt to reduce the hidden fat in your diet without losing the pleasure in your meals.

- Choose lean meats and trim all visible fat.
- Remove skin from chicken and other poultry.
- Avoid frying your food; instead try grilling, poaching, microwaving, braising or baking (be sure to place the meat on a rack standing in a pan containing water, not fat). If you do fry, use a non-stick pan and spray with a light mist of olive oil. Avoid deep-frying.
- Do not baste baked meat with fat or pan drippings; basting with wine or broth will keep the meat moist.
- Make soups or stews ahead of time and refrigerate overnight, then skim off the fat that hardens on top.
- When serving dips, swap high-fat potato chips and corn chips for julienne vegetables (carrots, capsicum and celery), for all the crunch without the kilojoules.
- Do you enjoy stir-fries? To reduce the quantity of oil required for stir-frying, use stock instead of oil or a non-stick wok.
- Spread butter or margarine thinly – it is easier if it is soft. Condiments (mustard, chutney, pickles) often make butter unnecessary for yummy sandwiches.
- A healthy alternative to sour cream on jacket potatoes is a dollop or two of plain low-fat yoghurt, cottage cheese or ricotta cheese.
- Avoid using breadcrumbs and flour, because they absorb more fat than if you simply sprayed the pan or used just a little oil. Schnitzels are loaded with fat!

- Use low/reduced-fat milk products.
- Do not slather cooked vegetables in butter — moisten them with homemade tomato sauce or lemon juice, and then garnish them with chopped parsley or chives. Use sauces (sweet chilli, soy, oyster) to add extra flavour.
- Slim down your salads. Salads will put you on the path to healthy eating, but beware of fatty dressing. If you spoon 4 tablespoons of full-fat dressing over your greens you may as well have consumed a cheeseburger. Use low-fat dressings, or dress your salad with balsamic vinegar, black pepper, lemon juice or a teaspoon of virgin olive oil and vinegar. Be careful of high-fat additions such as bacon bits, grated cheese and croutons.

Sugar

Sugar is empty kilojoules, so keep portions small, while enjoying the occasional treat. If you do have a sweet tooth, try these healthier, less kilojoule-laden options.

- Choose fresh fruits for desserts and snacks.
- Beware of hidden sugar in cordials, soft drinks, cakes, pastries and sweet biscuits. Limit your intake of chocolate, lollies and other sweets.
- Check the labels of your favourite foods — if sugar or sucrose is the first ingredient listed, the food is high in sugar.
- Do you have sugar in your tea or coffee? This can add up over a day! Try to cut back or eliminate sugar, or switch to artificial sweeteners.

Cookie cravings

Question: Sometimes I get major cravings for sweets and I eat packets of lollies or a box of chocolate biscuits. Why do I never crave apples or bananas?

Answer: Cravings usually come from being hungry, so snack regularly and don't skip meals. If you avoid becoming ravenous, you will have more restraint. Make sure your meals and snacks contain some protein and fat, which take longer to digest then carbohydrates and therefore help you feel satisfied for longer. You may also be turning to sweets simply because they are so readily available. Maintain a supply of fruit, cut-up veggies and wholemeal breads on hand, and ban biscuits from the house until you change your eating habits. For now, if you really want a biscuit or a piece of cake, create a situation where you have to go out and get it. Bananas and apples might seem less appealing to you than processed sweets, partly because you are not accustomed to eating fresh fruit. If you gradually cut back on added sugar you will eventually find that fruit hits the spot. Next time a craving hits, eat a piece of fruit and eventually this will become a habit — instead of just a sugar hit, you are treating your body to a feast of fibre, vitamins, minerals and phytochemicals.

Salt

Do you have a more savoury taste? You should not over-indulge in salt, because it can put you at risk of high blood pressure, stroke, cardiovascular disease or kidney disease. It can be difficult to know the quantity of added salt you are consuming, because there is a lot 'hidden' salt in processed foods such as bread, cheese, crackers, soups, stock cubes, yeast extract spreads and soy sauce, so check the labels. Salt is probably a habit you have acquired over a lifetime; if you cut back gradually, you will lose your taste for it. When preparing your food, consider the following tips.

- Do not put the saltshaker on the table.
- Do not add salt when cooking.
- Reduce your intake of processed, convenience and snack foods.
- Avoid very salty foods such as anchovies, salami, olives and potato crisps.
- Choose low salt or 'no added salt' products at the super-market.
- Use other condiments to enhance the flavour of foods.

SUMMING UP

∗ Meals must be tasty to be satisfying.
∗ Make every meal memorable with appealing flavours, textures and aromas.
∗ Learn to distinguish head and heart hunger from stomach hunger, and eat only when you are truly hungry. Ensure that what you eat is as appetising and tasty as possible.

Helen

Throughout most of my teenage years I wanted to lose weight. I would look at my friends, most of whom were naturally thin, and wished I could look like them in jeans or a bikini. I would start each year off and say to myself, 'This year I'm going to lose so much weight that people will actually start to notice.' So I would join a gym but rarely go, or go for a walk but only maybe once a month. When I was 14 and at a height of 162 centimetres I weighed approximately 70 kilograms – I felt awful. I barely had any confidence and it led to me feeling angry at myself for looking the way I did.

I had reached a point where no matter how hard I tried, I wasn't getting anywhere. I knew I wasn't eating badly, but no matter what I did I felt helpless – I didn't know why I wasn't losing weight. I really needed guidance on how to lose it properly and keep it off.

I started with Arlene when I was 17, and over the next year I dropped 12 kilograms. I realised that although I was eating relatively healthy foods, I was eating too much of those foods and at the wrong times. I learned how to eat properly, and not on a short-term basis, but every day. I never starve myself or deny my body protein or carbohydrates. I treat myself to chocolate and a scoop of ice-cream and it leaves me not wanting more. My mum always taught me that everything in moderation is okay; I just never did it.

Exercising every day also really helped me, not just because I was finally shedding kilos but because it lifted my mood and made me more able to work at school. By the end of the first month I was walking the same routes as I had in the beginning but in much less time. During the HSC, when everyone around me was putting on weight, I lost 8 kilograms. I discovered that you find your own rhythm, and everything becomes a habit. I only drink alcohol once or twice a month; I don't eat dinner late at night; and I avoid going out for pizza and pasta – not because I don't love pizza but because I know if I have one I will feel bloated and heavy the next day. I keep a bottle of water next to me all day and other than that I only drink Diet Coke. Being healthy and eating well makes me feel good, and that's why I do it.

My biggest temptation is lollies. I love the Natural Confectionery Company lollies, chocolate chip cookies and Crunchie Chocettes. Now I only indulge occasionally, but when I do I savour every second!

I go to the gym 3–4 times a week, and I walk every other day. I do cycle classes and Pilates, and I see a personal trainer who does weight training with me. Not only have I lost 12 kilograms, I have managed to keep that weight off, keep my body fit and toned and completely improve my lifestyle, mood and confidence. And now people notice I've lost weight.

CHAPTER **13**

THE NINTH COMMANDMENT:

Move it!

Exercise is one of the finest gifts you can give yourself. It is not only an essential weapon in your weight-loss arsenal, it has a host of other benefits. Prior to commencing any exercise regime you should consult your doctor.

Regular physical activity not only burns those excess kilojoules required for weight loss, it boosts your metabolic rate. Restricting your food intake can reduce your metabolic rate, making the exercise essential in helping compensate for this.

Exercise also helps you maintain muscle mass while you shed excess kilograms. If you lose weight by moderating your food intake alone, the loss of weight can be attributed to a 75 per cent loss of fat and 25 per cent loss of muscle. If you increase your exercise while eating less, you will lose the fat while maintaining your muscle mass.

When you have achieved your desired healthy weight, exercise becomes crucial in maintaining this new level. The vast majority of people who lose weight without working out, regain the kilos. Those who succeed in maintaining their healthy weight are those who take regular exercise.

In addition to helping you lose (and keep off) weight, exercise tones muscles, builds strength and flexibility, reduces blood pressure and cholesterol levels and helps prevent strokes, heart attacks and diabetes. Exercise also keeps bones healthy and helps prevent osteoporosis, boosts the immune system and may reduce the risk of certain types of cancer.

Have you ever noticed how exercise has a positive impact on your mood? Scientists studying the effect of exercise on mental wellbeing have found that it reduces anxiety and helps relieve or even prevent clinical depression. Exercise is a fantastic stress reliever and will motivate you to stick to your better eating plan. When you are feeling down in the dumps, head for the treadmill, not the fridge!

WHY DON'T WE EXERCISE?

Despite all the advantages of exercise, too many of us are just not active enough to experience the benefits. We are eating less than our ancestors, but we are also considerably less active, which is a major reason for the current epidemic of obesity afflicting Australia. How much less active? Well, a study conducted at Old Sydney Town (a replica of colonial Sydney that is now closed), monitored actors as they performed typical daily activities of the colonial era; the study showed that their efforts equated to the equivalent of walking 16 kilometres more a day than modern sedentary workers.

How exercise blasts fat

1. **It burns kilojoules.** A daily 30-minute brisk walk burns around 6300 kilojoules every week. Over six months this totals 163 800 kilojoules – the equivalent of over 5 kilograms of fat.

2. **It increases your metabolic rate.** Your metabolic rate stays elevated even after you've stopped exercising – the longer the duration or the more intense the exercise, the longer your metabolic rate remains elevated and the more kilojoules you burn. For example, after a 30-minute brisk walk, you burn an extra 210–336 kilojoules in recovery.

3. **It increases muscle tone.** Cutting down on kilojoules often produces loss of muscle, whereas exercise actually stimulates the release of growth hormones, which in turn stimulates the development of muscle tone.

4. **It makes you burn fat more efficiently.** During aerobic exercise your body produces hormones that activate the breakdown of stored fat to be used as fuel.

5. **It is an appetite suppressant.** A pre-lunch workout or walk can be very helpful in your weight-control plan. A walk after work is a great idea before sitting down to dinner – it allows you to unwind and reduces your hunger, allowing you to relax and enjoy your dinner and keep your portions moderate.

6. **It makes you fitter.** You will therefore be able to exercise for longer, burning more fat and more kilojoules.

How did we become so inactive? Modern conveniences play a prominent role, but the demands of earning a living make a huge contribution. Many people have office jobs, and sit the entire day. Working long hours, communicating via email, surfing the Internet and watching television without even having to rise from our chairs (courtesy of the remote control) all takes its toll.

Now, to the almighty automobile! Some people are so lazy that they are not prepared to walk so much as a block, but insist on parking right outside their destination. Result? Nil activity. It's a similar story with housework. Once, every-thing was done by hand, now we use labour-saving devices. In fact, it's been estimated that modern technology removes an average of 2100 kilojoules per week from our energy expenditure. That might not sound like much, but it equates to an extra 3.4 kilograms of fat over a year.

The bottom line: If you want to lose weight and keep it off, you must become more active. Remember this simple equa-tion: energy in (kilojoules) minus energy out (activity and metabolism) equals body weight. Increase the 'energy out' part of the equation, and you're well on your way to shedding the excess mass.

WHICH TYPE OF EXERCISE?

Any type – from lifting weights to swimming, dancing, play-ing tennis, running, walking, even running up stairs; just get moving. The best exercise is exercise you enjoy. If you like it, you'll do it regularly. One of my clients started belly dancing;

Question: I am 21, about 165 centimetres in height and weigh about 67 kilograms. This is the heaviest I have ever been and I am finding it really hard to lose weight due to just being too busy at work. I eat the right things but just can't get out to exercise. Any hints?

Answer: You have a BMI of 24.6, which falls within the healthy weight range. I understand you would like to be slimmer, but you have to remember a simple equation: energy in (kilojoules) minus energy out (activity and metabolism) will determine if you gain or lose weight. Consequently you will find it very difficult to lose weight without any exercise. In addition, muscle is more metabolically active than fat; you only build muscle tissue with exercise. Often during the day you might have ten minutes before work, ten minutes at lunchtime and ten minutes after work – try and utilise this time with a walk, and you are getting in 30 minutes of exercise during the day. Everyone has a few minutes in the day, which we spend on the phone, watching TV or socialising. Exercise with friends instead of going for coffee! Try and do high-quality and enjoyable activities/walks/gym sessions on the weekends. Watch your portion sizes and the foods you select.

she's 76, she loves it and it's keeping her in great shape!

There are three components to exercise, important individually and in combination. Ideally, your exercise regime should involve all three.

- **Cardiovascular.** Cardiovascular workouts – which include activities such as brisk walking, jogging, running, aerobics or swimming – increase the heart rate to strengthen the heart muscle.
- **Strength training.** Strength training strengthens the muscles by working against resistance, such as with steppers, rowing machines, weights and elastic exercise bands.
- **Flexibility training.** This increases the elasticity of the muscles and enhances the way they work together.

HOW MUCH EXERCISE?

Aim to exercise for at least 45 minutes a day, every day. More is better. People often remark they can't possibly fit a whole 45 minutes of exercise into their busy schedule. Break it up into manageable short stints – for example, 15 minutes before work, 15 minutes at lunchtime and 15 minutes after work. Everyone has a few minutes spare in the day, which they spend watching TV, on the telephone or simply doing nothing. Why not use that time to do push-ups on the kitchen counter, leg extensions while sitting in a chair, or lunges and squats, using soup cans as weights?

PLAN YOUR PROGRAM

Don't make the mistake of thinking that you can be sedentary all week and make up for it on the weekend. Weekend exercisers must make time in their daily schedules for exercise, because a little every day is better than a lot occasionally.

Question: How long should I exercise for to lose weight? I only enjoy walking. At the moment I am walking four times a week for half an hour. Is this enough?

Answer: Losing weight is dependent on energy balance – the amount of food you consume versus the energy your body utilises. When you burn more energy than you eat, you will lose weight. For years it was recommended that you should do 30 minutes of exercise each day, but the recommendation is changing to 60 minutes of moderately intense activity (such as brisk walking) each day. I suggest you do as much as your schedule allows – but make exercise a priority. The amount of exercise you should do also depends on how sedentary you are the rest of the day. I suggest you aim for an hour's walk each day, and on the days you cannot manage the full hour, try and walk at a faster pace.

Start by setting realistic goals, particularly if you are unfit. Instead of jumping right into a strenuous jogging program – which is bound to exhaust or injure you – start with walking, increase your session by an extra five minutes every third day and slowly increase the pace, then eventually alternate 10 minutes of jogging with 10 minutes of walking, and so on. Try to do a little more each time and vary your activities as you increase them; you could add a 20-minute weight training session three times a week, cycling to work, taking a salsa class or even skipping with your children.

Results come with persistence, so it is essential to persevere! I guarantee that once you establish an exercise habit, you'll start to enjoy it and depend on it. Track your efforts in an exercise diary so you can appreciate your accomplishments – here's an example to get you started.

Your seven-day exercise diary

MONDAY [DATE]

activity _____

duration _____

intensity _____

TUESDAY [DATE]

activity _____

duration _____

intensity _____

WEDNESDAY [DATE]

activity _____

duration _____

intensity _____

THURSDAY [DATE]

activity _____

duration _____

intensity _____

FRIDAY [DATE]

activity _____

duration _____

intensity _____

SATURDAY [DATE]

activity _____

duration _____

intensity _____

SUNDAY [DATE]

activity _____

duration _____

intensity _____

WHEN'S THE RIGHT TIME?

When is the best time to exercise? It's up to you; work out when it best suits your schedule. Your metabolism accelerates after your exercise session, and this occurs no matter when you do the workout. The additional kilojoule burn is related to how long and how hard you have worked out, not the time of day.

That said, it is true that morning exercisers tend to have more success sticking to their activity schedules, simply because obstacles can pile up during the course of the day. However, some people struggle to get up early in the morning. I am a morning person, and I prefer to exercise before breakfast;

I always walk before I eat. Physiologically it is better to exercise before you have eaten, because you will burn fat as a source of energy rather than the glucose you have just consumed.

It is more important to establish a regular pattern of exercise than to worry about what time of day it occurs. Think of it this way: the best time for exercising is your worst time for eating. Many mothers tend to overeat in the afternoon, when their children come home from school. If that sounds like you, why not take the children to play in the park instead of snacking at home all afternoon? People

> *'You have to stay in shape. My grandmother, she started walking 5 miles a day when she was 60. She's 97'*
>
> ❧
>
> ELLEN DeGENERES

who have been working all day often cannot stop eating when they get home, and then graze in front of the television after dinner. To prevent this, a session of exercise when you return home will relax you and cease the pre-dinner snacking, or a walk as soon as you have finished dinner will put a stop to eating in front of the television.

HOW HARD?

What aerobic intensity is most effective in burning fat? You should aim to exercise at 60–80 per cent of your maximum heart rate. How do you calculate this? Subtract your age from 220, then multiply first by 0.6 then by 0.8 to find the correct range. For example, a 34-year-old would be between 112 and 150 beats per minute. You can also judge your effort level. On a scale of 1 to 10 (1 being sitting, 10 an all-out sprint); you should strive for 6–8. When you work out at this pace, at least half your fuel comes from body fat.

A simpler way of gauging exercise intensity is to apply the 'talk test': if you can talk while exercising without puffing, you are working out at the right level. If you can't speak without gasping for breath, reduce your effort until you can talk comfortably.

UPPING THE ANTE

Some people find that they've stopped losing weight, despite faithfully performing the same amount of exercise. This is due to their muscles becoming accustomed to the same workout, which results in the workout becoming less effective. Your body is designed to be as energy-efficient as possible. As your muscles adapt to your exercise regime you burn fewer kilojoules. There are ways to overcome this. Begin by gradually increasing the intensity of your workout. If you normally walk for 45 minutes, increase your speed so that you're clocking the same distance in 40 minutes, and in the extra 5 minutes you can extend the distance of your walk or do a sprint or jog. Start adding sprints and alternate three minutes of running with three minutes of walking. Include some hills in your route, which will force your muscles to work harder and burn more kilojoules.

Finally, there's cross-training (varying your activities) to keep your muscles from becoming accustomed to any one

Why not walk?

Walking is something we do every day; don't underestimate the value of it. It is one of the best forms of exercise you can do for overall fitness, because it uses nearly all the muscles of the body. Walking is a weight-bearing exercise, which means that it is more strenuous than you might imagine. At the same time, it is low impact, which means it's safer for your back and joints than other forms of exercise involving jumping or impacting your knees, hips and ankles. How much walking is best? Aim for 10 000 steps (7–8 kilometres, depending on the length of your stride) a day. Here are some tips to get you started.

- Wear supportive shoes, a hat and sunscreen.
- Start with a 10–20-minute walk every day, and then gradually work up to 45 minutes or more.
- Commence each walk slowly and then increase the pace. Aim for a pace that leaves you slightly breathless but still able to carry on a conversation.
- Swing your arms and hold your head high, your shoulders back, your chest lifted and your stomach pulled in.
- Keep track of your progress with a pedometer, a device worn on your waistband (available at sports stores or gyms) that measures steps taken, distance covered and sometimes even kilojoules burned.
- To avoid dehydration, drink water during and after walking, especially in hot weather.

exercise. Twice a week, replace your walk with a 45-minute bike ride, boxing, dance class or other activity.

SEEK SUPPORT

Getting fit is a long-term objective, so it's important to surround yourself with positive people who will help keep you motivated. Forget the mates who urge you to skip your workouts and go to the pub for a drink instead. Rather, picture your wife's pleasure as your fitness improves, or your boyfriend's smile when he sees you in that slinky dress that fits again thanks to your workouts. The support of people who care about you will help keep you on track to achieve your exercise goals. Often people find that exercise is their 'time out', when they want to switch off and have no-one around.

KEEPING IT UP

You don't have to remind yourself to brush your teeth every day – it's a learned habit. Exercise will also become an entrenched habit if you do it regularly and keep yourself motivated. These tips will help.

- Be prepared. Make each exercise session as effortless as possible by packing your gym gear the night before and having it ready by the front door.
- Make it a group effort. Working out by yourself can become lonely and boring. Involving others can help keep you on track. Jog with friends, take a class at the gym, and don't forget to include your pet – walking the dog isn't just good for the dog, it's good for you.

Excuses, excuses

Here are four commonly cited obstacles to exercise and how to overcome them.

1. I don't have the time

- Exercise first thing in the morning before other obligations intrude.
- Combine activities, such as riding your bike to work or holding 'walking meetings' with colleagues. Do errands – such as shopping or banking – on foot or by bike.

2. It's cold and wet outside

- Find indoor options: home equipment, exercise videos, television workout shows.
- Invest in sports clothing suitable for working out in wet, cold or hot weather.

3. I'm too tired

- Recruit an exercise buddy to keep you motivated.
- Work out early. If you plan to exercise after work, have an energising snack mid-afternoon.

4. I don't have childcare

- If you work outside the home, exercise during your lunch break.
- Take the kids with you. Put the baby in a jogging stroller. Bike or hike with older children. Why not kick a ball around the park together? Beats slumping on the couch watching cartoons with them!
- Use the indoor options listed above.

- Set short-term goals – such as working out every day for a fortnight – and reward yourself when you reach them. Give yourself non-food treats such as a massage or a new CD.

AND REMEMBER . . .

Changing your lifestyle doesn't just apply to the way you eat and exercise. It includes actively seeking to relax and be happy. Too many people suffer from stress, which can manifest itself in overeating, headaches, constipation and feelings of tension. They often say they are too busy to squeeze anything more into their hectic schedules, let alone take regular exercise. Does that sound like you? If so, make time to relax, otherwise it is difficult to enjoy anything in your daily activities.

The true measure of fitness isn't how far you can run or how many sit-ups you can do. A truly fit person makes an effort to balance every aspect of life, not just exercise. You make eating well a priority. You enjoy your job and have a positive outlook on life. You get pleasure from exercising and enjoy the benefits you experience from it. You relax and enjoy recreation, family and social time. Once you recognise how crucial every aspect of your life is in terms of your overall health and fitness, you start to realise your full potential. When you've struck a balance between all these elements, you can label yourself truly fit.

Burn 500 kilojoules fast!

Here are ten quick ways to burn 500 kilojoules*. Put several of the points listed below together into one intense workout, or spread them throughout your day. The more you do, the more kilojoules you burn and the faster your metabolic rate. If you do just four exercise hits a day, you can shed over 1 kilogram of fat a month!

1. **Run up stairs for 8½ minutes**

   Turn the stairs at home or work into an in-house 'gym', or find a steep hill to tackle on your regular running route. Only count the time spent going up, and always walk – don't run – down stairs, to safeguard your knees.

2. **Skip for 12 minutes**

   If you are adept at fancy footwork, add this to your workout by hopping on one foot, twisting from side to side, or moving around the room as you skip. Increase the intensity by jumping twice per second.

3. **Run for 15 minutes**

   If you run 1.5 kilometres in 10 minutes, you'll burn approximately 500 kilojoules in 15 minutes. Increase your speed by pumping your arms as you run.

4. **Cycle for 20 minutes**

   Aim for 22–25 kilometres-per-hour or a pace where you are working fairly hard.

5. Yoga for 25 minutes

Power (Asthanga) yoga – which involves switching postures frequently, as opposed to just holding one pose and meditating – builds muscular endurance while it stretches your muscles. The more vigorous the postures, the more kilojoules you'll zap.

6. Circuit train for 13 minutes

Circuit training involves progressing from one gym machine 'station' to another without resting. For example, you do 15 reps on the leg-extension machine, immediately jump on the squat-press machine, then progress to the calf-raise station and so on. Many gyms set up their machines in an easy-to-follow circuit format, or you can take a circuit class.

7. Callisthenics for 15 minutes

Push-ups, sit-ups, jumping jacks and squats are great kilojoule burners as well as strengtheners.

8. Power walk for 15 minutes

Keep up a good pace (you want to cover 1 kilometre in 8–10 minutes). Speed it up by pumping your arms and pushing off with the toes of your rear foot.

9. Rollerblade for 10 minutes

A great workout – and fun too!

10. Weight train for 20 minutes (with heavier weights; 35 minutes with lighter weights)

The heavier the weights (appropriate to your size and strength), the more muscle mass you will build, and the greater the boost to your metabolic rate, which will result in burning more kilojoules.

*All kilojoule counts are approximate for a 60-kilogram woman. (For men: I always say that it's a man's world – if you weigh more you will burn more.)

SUMMING UP

✱ Increasing your physical activity is essential to attaining and maintaining a healthy weight. Exercise speeds your metabolism. It also lifts your mood and reduces the risk of cardiovascular disease, diabetes and other diseases.

✱ Aim for at least 45 minutes of exercise a day. Set realistic goals and gradually build up your activity level, both in time and intensity.

✱ Plan your exercise program to fit into your daily schedule. Keep a diary of your efforts to monitor your progress.

✱ Choose a form of exercise that you enjoy, and you are more likely to do it. Walking is easy to fit into a business schedule.

✱ Exercise in company – this will encourage you and keep you moving on days when your motivation flags.

SUCCESS *Tricia* STORY

I first went to see Arlene eighteen months after the birth of my second child. I had become lazy in my eating habits and even lazier in my exercise routine. During my early twenties I had been slim and could eat what I wanted without a specific exercise plan and still maintain my figure. As I moved into my thirties this changed, and once I had children the problem worsened. As a working mother I was eating too much takeaway food and snacking constantly. Then my mother told me that she had put on over 6 kilograms with each of her three children, and she had not lost any of the weight. I did not want to repeat that. I went on a family holiday with friends and was too embarrassed to be seen in my swimming costume. This meant I could not properly enjoy myself and play with my kids by the pool. I knew I had to make changes and make them now. Four months later I had lost 17 kilograms and was weighing less than I had when I got married eight years previously.

The first thing I did was reassess my portions, and I stopped snacking between meals. I did not 'cut out' anything from my diet; I just reduced it to a sensible amount. I made sure I had a good-sized, healthy breakfast, and I reduced my dinners considerably. I also tried to walk for at least an hour every day. Previously, exercise had been something I would avoid at all costs, but once I started walking I couldn't stop. The best part of it was that I invited a few girlfriends to join me, so it became a social event as well as a health issue. As a very busy working mother with two children, I came to value the time I walked to catch up with my friends or just listen to my walkman and have some time to myself. I found that if I didn't walk for a day or so I missed it, and I now feel calmer at home because of it – it helps release a lot of frustration at the end of the day!

The important thing I have learned is that you should not deprive yourself of anything. If you do, you eat more of something else to compensate. Have what you want in moderation and ensure that you expend more or equal energy to what you consume. If you are going out and want to indulge – do an extra walk and enjoy both the meal and the exercise.

CHAPTER 14

THE TENTH COMMANDMENT:

Balance your life

Balancing your life is imperative for achieving success in any undertaking. Without balance in your life, you will have great difficulty achieving a healthy eating and exercising pattern. By 'balance', I mean acknowledging the importance of your personal as well as your professional life; and giving the appropriate weight and time to your relationships, rewarding activities and pleasurable pastimes, as well as to your paid work.

Sounds simple, but balance is something so many of us fail to achieve. Some time ago I met a senior executive who gave his office as his home address, so I asked if he lived in the city. He replied, no, and that his home was in the suburbs, but that his family always told him that he 'lived' at work, because he was always there. He never came home in time for dinner, he had no time for exercise, no time to socialise or spend time with his family. He did not just live *at* work, he lived *for* work. He believed he had no time for anything else.

I told him that unless he learned to balance his life, he was going to continue missing out on so much.

I get caught in this trap. Work could consume my life if I allowed it, because I am a career woman as well as a mother. I try to balance my life so that I can enjoy a family life with my children, earn a living, socialise, run a home and have time to exercise. I know how much you lose if you work too hard because I have seen how stressed I become if I take on too much. I try and make time for all the other things that are important to me.

> '*Success is not final, failure is not fatal: it is the courage to continue that counts*'
>
> WINSTON CHURCHILL

I derive great pleasure from spending time with my children, I have fun being with my partner and I also like being alone to recharge my batteries. No matter how busy I am, I make time to prepare a meal, eat with my family and take a walk each day. There are other activities that make life more enjoyable – having your hair done, a manicure, a massage, a movie, reading or playing bridge – and it is very important to make time to partake in everything in moderation.

Balancing your life means putting yourself first. There is more to life than work, rush and stress. Yet some people are so busy they forget. This is when food can become their only friend, and consequently their weight is affecting their life. Some people do not relax; in fact, some fear relaxation, and feel guilty when they do nothing. They cannot unwind, because they have been so busy making a living or looking after the home that they have forgotten how to make a life. They use food as a tranquiliser.

Does this sound familiar? If you feel your life is unbalanced, remember that it is important to schedule fun into your life, just as you now make time for work, children or perhaps studies. Take a few moments to consider what you enjoy doing – it might be doing a crossword, bushwalking, taking an art class or simply chilling out doing nothing at all. It is well worth the investment of your time if it is calming and good for your mood.

How are you spending your time?

Estimate how many minutes per day you spend on the following activities, and how long you would like to spend. In the third box calculate how much time you could realistically spend on these activities without causing too much disruption to your schedule. Be realistic. I am certain that you can accumulate at least 30 minutes from your workday or home chores to devote to other, more fulfilling activities . . . and this is a fundamental step towards restoring important balance to your life.

Activity	Time you spend now	Time you would like to spend	Time you could spend
Working			
Sleeping			
Travelling to and from work			
Shopping			
Cooking			
Eating			
Talking to your partner			
Playing with the kids			
Sport or exercise			
Keeping in touch with friends and relatives			
Playing with pet/s			
On the computer			
Crafts and hobbies			
Listening to music			
Reading			
Watching television			
Self-care (grooming, etc)			
Prayer, meditation, religious activity			
Education			
Enjoying nature			
Helping others			
Other activities (specify)			

Add up the totals. There are no correct or incorrect answers, but if there is a big discrepancy between the figure in the left-hand box and the other two, it could be time to consider ways of bringing more balance into your life. Try changing one thing – for example, finish work 20 minutes earlier so you can spend time with your family. Once you have started making changes, it will be easier to make others. The first step is to identify what needs to be changed, then to focus on small and achievable ways of making these adjustments.

BEATING THE WORK BANDWAGON

It is easy to get onto the bandwagon of work or a frenzied lifestyle; once aboard, you go faster and faster, and it is difficult to get off – until you get a wake-up call. It might be a medical check-up, a heart attack, rising cholesterol or blood sugar or other warning sign that your way of life is impacting your health. Only then do you wake up and take notice. I meet many people in this situation – they are referred to me by their doctor. They want advice on losing weight, on controlling their diabetes or another nutritional issue. The primary action I tell them to take is to balance their lives.

How easy is this to achieve? It can be hard, but often simple changes will put you on the correct path. A senior manager told me that the greatest thing I did for her was suggest she go for a walk first thing each morning. She was stressed, working long hours, and it had never occurred to her that walking was an easy, low-tech way to de-stress and boost her health. Now she arrives at the office half-an-hour later than previously, but the company is surviving and she is thriving. She recently purchased a treadmill so that she could weather a storm. She has realised that she *can* change her life.

BUT I HAVE TO WORK THIS HARD!

Overworking is not always a matter of choice. The reality is that many people work increasingly long hours because they feel insecure both financially and in their job. This makes it difficult to object to working longer hours when the person in charge expects you to work unpaid overtime. Consider the following: if you are hired to work from 9 to 5 and you are regularly working until 6, 7 or even later each night, you are giving the company a bonus of 5, 10 or more hours a week. That is the equivalent of over a day's work that they are not paying for per week! Is that fair or reasonable? No. Can you maintain this? You are setting standards that will be expected of you in the future, while the quality of your life is suffering.

Do you want to continue living like this? If the answer is no, what can you do about it? Be assertive, but pleasant. Explain to your superior that the hours you are working are unsustainable and that the quality of your work will suffer because you are exhausted and stressed. Attempt to strike a balance: you are prepared to work until 6 in emergencies, but not on a regular basis. You will then arrive home in time for dinner with your family.

What are the most central things in your life? Generally they are your relationships with family and friends. How much time are you devoting to these people? Many Australians are opting for 'voluntary simplicity', in which they scale down their material requirements, choosing to work less and enjoy the important things in life more – spending time with loved ones, learning new skills and pursuing interests. Does that sound appealing? Can you make it happen for you?

> *'Life wasn't meant to be easy – but take courage . . . because it can be delightful'*
>
> — GEORGE BERNARD SHAW

If you had six months to live, what would you do? Continue your current existence without change, or would you try to do all the things you have always wanted to do but put off because there was always something more urgent demanding your attention? I am not the first person to recommend that you live and enjoy every day of your life. Nobody ever died wishing they had spent more time working, but there are a lot of people who die wishing that they had not. Do not become one of them.

BEATING BURNOUT

Many of us feel we have no escape but to continue coping with work, family and financial problems. Eventually the stress over weeks, months and years results in a wasted life. Unless you take measures to enjoy each day, you will suffer burnout.

Burnout is a state of utter mental and physical exhaustion

Anthony, 35, accountant

Anthony was employed by a leading auditing firm. He was working 12-hour days, which meant that he missed out on spending time with his wife and their two daughters. He had no time for playing sport, which he had always enjoyed, and he had become pudgy and unfit. His workload increased after the firm retrenched several senior accountants in order to reduce costs. Exhausted, Anthony put in a leave form, planning a family holiday. The firm agreed — subject to his taking his laptop and continuing to meet his weekly deadlines. The break was disastrous: all work and very little play. The experience woke him up to how out of kilter his life had become. He told his manager that he would now leave the office by 6 p.m. He joined a soccer team. His superior was furious, as Anthony had anticipated. Anthony had already made contacts, and within a month he was offered a job at a less-demanding firm. Now Anthony is trimmer and happier. He has more time for other activities and his family — and a more balanced life.

that leaves you feeling drained, alienated and unproductive. Easy tasks become difficult or impossible to accomplish. Worst of all, you no longer care. This can happen to any-one — mothers, fathers, teenagers, professionals, labourers. If your life is not in balance and you are not feeling fulfilled and content, depression can set in.

In order to combat burnout, consider these tips.

- Take a break. Look at matters objectively and ascertain what you want in the long term. Do you really need that new car, computer or holiday home? How far do you want to go in your career, and what are you prepared to sacrifice to achieve it? Is your present way of life the one you truly want or just the way things seem to have turned out?

- Learn to say no. Be assertive, manage your time and perhaps take classes in negotiation skills. Many community colleges offer courses in these techniques; check your library or bookshop for books on these topics.

- Visualisation – mentally picture yourself coping in different situations. It increases your sense of control, which is vital for combatting stress.

- Look after yourself. If you get enough sleep, stop smoking, control alcohol consumption, exercise regularly and eat correctly, you will be in better shape to cope with all the competing demands.

- Exercise daily. This gives your mind a break, helping you get rid of stress and frustration.

- Share your problems with people you trust, expressing your feelings calmly and non-judgementally. Talking to others is often therapeutic.

- Practice relaxation and meditation techniques to help ease the burden of stress.

Seven ways to stress less

Stress has myriad physical and psychological effects. It goes directly to your stomach. It leads to both irritable bowel syndrome (nervous indigestion, bloating, constipation, diarrhoea) and abdominal fat around your middle that can be very hard to budge. That is because fat in the abdominal area functions differently than fat elsewhere in your body. It has a greater blood supply and more receptors for cortisol, a stress hormone. Cortisol levels rise and fall throughout the day, but when you are under constant stress, levels remain elevated.

With continuing high stress and, consequently, high cortisol levels, more fat gets deposited in the abdominal area where there are more cortisol receptors. This is

dangerous because abdominal fat – or central obesity – is associated with higher rates of cardiovascular disease, type 2 diabetes and several types of cancer.

Abdominal fat is not the only price to pay for chronic stress. Chronically high cortisol levels interfere with the production of feel-good neuro-transmitters – such as dopamine and serotonin – which can lead to depression and you feeling more stressed. The cycle repeats itself. Unchecked stress can lead to health and marital problems, trouble with children and even death.

Losing weight is not the only answer. Research indicates that if stress levels remain high, abdominal fat will increase even if your body is lean elsewhere. People called 'high-stress responders' (those who secrete more cortisol in response to stress), have more central fat, regardless of their overall body fat.

Certain changes to your food intake could help you combat abdominal fat. The Mediterranean diet – high in fish, nuts, seeds, whole grains, beans, fruits and vegetables – appears to have an anti-inflammatory effect on the body, helping fight the damaging effects of chronic stress. The nutrients showing the most promise for long-term stress relief are omega-3 fatty acids, the keystone of the Mediterranean diet. These are healthy fats found in oily fish such as salmon, herring, sardines and mackerel, and also in flaxseed and nuts. As odd as it may sound, getting more of these 'good' fats is associated with reduction in body fat, including dangerous abdominal fat. They can also reduce the output of another stress hormone, epinephrin (adrenaline).

While experts do know that high cortisol levels contribute to abnormal accumulation of abdominal fat and the subsequent development of life-threatening diseases, they have not yet come up with a magic nail to permanently deflate your spare tyre. Adopting habits such as regular exercise and relaxation techniques are the keys to creating a healthy, happy life. If you want to get rid of abdominal fat, start relaxing. Here are seven useful stress-reduction techniques for you to try.

1. Breath control

Many of us overbreathe when stressed, leading to feelings of breathlessness and panic.

Slow down by practising this simple exercise. Close your eyes and breathe in slowly through your nose, concentrating on filling your abdomen rather than your chest with air. Now slowly exhale while mentally saying the word 'relax'. Repeat this whenever you are feeling rushed or flustered.

2. Progressive relaxation

This means systematically relaxing every muscle in turn. Lie comfortably on your back on the floor. Clench and then relax your right foot, then your right leg, then the right side of your chest and abdomen, and then your right hand, arm and shoulder. Repeat for your left side. Finish with your face, paying attention to the muscles around your eyes and mouth.

3. Yoga

Yoga combines controlled breathing, meditation and gentle stretching to calm the mind and strengthen the body.

4. Tai Chi

Tai Chi requires deep concentration while practising slow, rhythmic movements. It promotes relaxation by aligning the body so that the muscles are in perfect balance.

5. Meditation

This involves focusing on a single image or sound – perhaps a mantra (a word repeated over and over) or the sound of your own breathing. This calms the mind by clearing it of random thoughts. Classes in meditation as well as Tai Chi, yoga and relaxation are widely available; check your local paper, community health centre, library bulletin board, the Internet or the *Yellow Pages* for details.

6. Massage

Massage – rhythmic kneading and stroking of the major muscle groups – is soothing. There are many forms of massage, including shiatsu (involving pressure applied along the body's meridians) and reflexology (pressure applied to points on the feet) and aromatherapy (using different oils for tranquility, stress relief and relaxation).

7. Time out

Try to factor frequent breaks into your routine. Take your allotted holidays, and indulge in weekends away whenever you can. Plan a few hours to indulge yourself to recharge your batteries. Regular exercise is therapeutic; a daily 45-minute walk, swim or any other activity you enjoy will soak up stress.

THE POWER OF POTTERING

Fulfilling activities bring pleasure and meaning to your life. Many of these are relaxing, but not all relaxing activities are considered productive. Some may seem quite mundane: pottering around the house or garden, or simply doing nothing. Unfortunately, these pastimes, which can be soothing and restorative, are often the first casualties of overwork, having children, or generally living a frenzied life. Do not underestimate their power; if they help you combat stress, they are worthwhile. Here is a list of activities many people find relaxing. Highlight those you most enjoy and keep the list handy to remind yourself to indulge as often as possible.

Having a bath or shower	Going for a drive
Watching television	Window-shopping
Listening to the radio	Gardening
Going to the movies	Tinkering in the shed
Chatting on the phone to friends	Washing your car
Rearranging the furniture or sorting your drawers	Going to the park
	Sitting in the sun
Reading a novel or magazine	Add suggestions of your own:
Playing cards or a board game	_____
Doing your hair or nails	_____
Visiting the library	_____

GETTING THERE

You must continually work to achieve balance in your life. Our lives are forever experiencing change, and we need to adapt. You have to persevere in making time for yourself, others and work. When you are more balanced you will feel less anxious and more energetic, you will no longer feel that there are not enough hours in the day to fulfill all your obligations, and you will stop automatically reaching for food to calm you down. You will notice the positive flow-on effects on your weight and general wellbeing – which makes the effort worthwhile.

SUMMING UP

* In order to balance your eating, you must first balance your life.
* Try to work out ways to achieve a desirable equilibrium between your professional, domestic and personal requirements.

✱ Consider activities you find rewarding, fulfilling or just plain fun, and make more time for them.

SUCCESS *Kayla* STORY

I grew up in a large, wonderful family with energetic brothers who had big appetites, and a gorgeous mum who always cooked delicious meals and treats. Fortunately the yummy food was never a major issue, because we were always running around, swimming and playing.

It wasn't until my early twenties when I got my first office job that I really started to gain weight. I was working long hours in a stressful environment and sitting at a desk all day – everyone always had lollies and chocolates, and we'd nibble a lot. I'd often go drinking after work with colleagues and clients, and it was easy to grab takeaway for dinner rather than cooking at home. I thought I never had time for exercise, because I was working such long hours. I'd eat out a few nights a week with my boyfriend, and we would always share a bottle of wine and have dessert . . . Three years later, I'd piled on the kilos. I was very unhappy with my appearance and it was frustrating, because I had always been an active person and now I felt it was beyond me.

When the relationship ended I was very upset. It was the turning point for me. I was angry with myself for putting on weight. I felt ugly and my clothes didn't fit, so I decided to do something about it. I'd heard of this scary, strict diet guru, and I knew that if I wanted to do this properly I should go and see her. Well . . . I walked out of my first appointment in complete shock. She'd told me that 'yes' I was fat and 'yes' I did need to lose weight. No sympathy! I suppose she just told me the truth, and it was hard to hear. But my stubborn Taurus determination and willpower came out and I was determined to be her best student!

Every Tuesday I'd weigh in, and I started getting results. It wasn't rocket science, it was a lifestyle change. I walked for an hour every day and made it a priority. I reduced my alcohol intake. I learned about portion sizes, fresh fruit and vegetables and generally how to 'think like a thin person'. Arlene was encouraging, but also extremely strict with me and never let me fall off the rails two weeks in a row.

I started seeing a great guy who is very loving, supportive and also physically active. Together we began exercising on weekends and before or after work. The motivation and dedication needs to come from yourself, but it makes it so much easier if your other half understands and assists in achieving your goals. I now had a new goal . . . I wanted to look good not just for me, but for him! I was spurred on every time I got dressed to go out and he showered me with compliments and told me how much he loved hanging off my arm at parties.

I'm now much happier and feel I have reclaimed my health and feeling of self-worth.

I have a great balance between work, play and exercise. Life is not always easy, but it's important to keep a positive attitude, because you *can* achieve whatever you set your mind to.

CHAPTER 15

Staying on track

You are finally at your goal weight! How do you know? Because when your body reaches the weight it is comfortable with, you will stay at this level. Now what? It is normal to slip up occasionally. If, however, these overindulgences become too frequent, you need to take action and control. A bad day at work or a stressful social situation, and it seems that only a generous serve of fudge cake can soothe your soul. One kilo creeps on, then another, and before you know it, your weight is right back to where it started.

Many people who successfully lose weight eventually regain it. You *must* break this relapse cycle. Forget the past, and embrace your new lifestyle. Remember the First Commandment? You are not on a diet, you have adopted a new lifestyle; your eating plan and exercise regime are forever. You must accept this new approach as 'normal' life — there is no deprivation to endure, because there is nothing you cannot eat, as long as you watch your portion sizes and balance your eating and activity level. It is imperative to weigh yourself regularly, so you are aware of any weight gain or loss and can adjust your portion size and exercise routine accordingly.

Maintaining a healthy weight is a lifelong commitment – enough hopping on and off the diet carousel. You must beat the statistics and avoid reverting to unhealthy behaviour patterns. You obviously had a clear idea of what you wanted to achieve in terms of losing weight and increasing your fitness, or you would not have continued reading to this page.

Why is it so tough to maintain a healthier lifestyle? It is a huge challenge to maintain new patterns forever. The change from 'diet' to 'lifestyle' can be extremely hard to make. When you have a goal to achieve, it is easy to remain motivated, but after you have achieved your objective you cannot continue feeling that same level of motivation. You now have to accept that an improved lifestyle needs constant discipline until it becomes a habit. When you are feeling tired or unhappy, it is easy to take the lazy option – become a couch potato enjoying chips, biscuits, lollies, chocolate or ice-cream in front of the television in preference to taking an after-dinner walk. Once you start relapsing, it is essential to recognise that you are reverting to old patterns that have been ingrained for many years. Habits are like creases in a sheet of paper: once they are there they keep falling into the same folds and can be hard to eradicate. You must stay positive and persevere; old habits *can* be replaced with healthier new ones for the long term.

Losing weight is hard work; keeping it off requires

continual vigilance. You must be aware of your food choices and portion sizes, and monitor your behaviour to ensure that you do not slip back into your old habits. Remember the techniques you have learned to cope with loneliness, boredom and other negative emotions without turning to food. Identify your danger zones (times of day, certain situations or particular people) and plan strategies to avoid or defuse them. Remember, exercise is a great stress reliever!

Whenever you feel yourself wavering from your new routine, consider the potential consequences. Do you want to gain weight? Remember how you felt when you were overweight? How you looked? (Looking at a photograph is a quick reminder.) Consider how you will feel when you drink or eat too much – is the instant gratification worth the long-term problems you will suffer? I don't think so, and I don't think you do either, or you would not have gone to all the effort in the first place. Whenever temptation strikes, stop, relax and take the time to make an objective decision that you will not regret. Never argue with yourself – Should I skip my walk today? Should I eat that extra biscuit? – or you are already halfway on the road to collapse. Make no exceptions or your resolve will quickly unravel and the exception will become the rule. Only eat when you are relaxed, the food is on a plate and you are sitting down – your eating will otherwise be unrestrained.

Continually reinforce your will to succeed by treating yourself with non-food rewards whenever you have achieved a goal. Feeling great is a reward in itself!

Question: I have lost a lot of weight over the past two years but I still have another 5 kilograms to go. The trouble is that I get so tired that I find it hard to stay motivated. Any ideas to help me get my energy back?

Answer: I can understand that you feel frustrated at not shifting those final 5 kilograms, but you should be proud of yourself for having been successful in losing so many kilos so far. Having shed this excess, you should now feel full of energy. Perhaps you have eliminated certain foods from your diet and are now missing out on some of your nutrient requirements. Consult your doctor to investigate your ongoing fatigue, because it could be a symptom of a problem such as anaemia (lack of iron), depression, a sleep disorder, over-exercising, thyroid abnormality or inappropriate eating patterns. Are you eating a balanced diet? Be careful not to starve yourself and omit essential nutrients, because this will sap your energy and harm your health. Include some lean red meat in your diet, along with plenty of fruit, vegetables and grains, and make sure your fluid intake is sufficient to remain hydrated. Each day eat three small meals and three snacks to avoid fluctuations in blood glucose levels, and exercise for 45 minutes. Not only should your energy return, so should your motivation.

Forgive yourself the odd hiccup, provided these do not become too frequent.

Strengthen your resolve by regularly reviewing each of the 10 Commandments whenever your motivation flags.

ARE YOU BEING UNDERMINED?

Often the problem is not only maintaining your own motivation but also coping with people's reaction to the new, attractive, healthy and slimmer you. Unfortunately, it is frequently people you expected to applaud your efforts and achievement who now appear to be sabotaging you. Consider Cassie, 42, who finally succeeded in losing the excess weight that had depressed her for so many years, only to find that her relationship with supposedly supportive friends had deteriorated. 'One friend was particularly nasty and I felt so hurt,' said Cassie. 'We started exercising and watching our food together, but Pam gave up when I did not. Now she is making me feel bad about losing the weight. Is this normal behaviour?'

Unfortunately, it is. Losing weight can impact friendships and relationships. True friends should be delighted with your achievements. Cassie's friend is obviously envious of her success and frustrated by her own failure. Family members, and even partners, can react in surprising ways when you start to make positive changes to your life. The tall poppy syndrome is prevalent; your improvements might make people around you feel vulnerable and insecure, or even affect their self-esteem. Perhaps they recognise their inadequacy when you are positive and self-confident, feeling and looking great.

There are numerous approaches to dealing with the

situation. Do not let these people undermine you, because regaining those lost kilos will not rectify the relationships. Taking the line of least resistance might make life seem easier now, but ultimately the resentment that it generates will drive a wedge between you. Rather, confront friends or relatives who are treating you differently since you lost weight and ask them why the relationship has changed. Explain that you still love and care for them and that you need their support. Try to understand their behaviour, and reassure them that even though your figure and lifestyle might have improved, you are the same person – your feelings and personality are identical. If you do not get the support you need, it is time to re-evaluate the relationship. Spend time with people who support you and have a positive influence in your life.

OVERCOMING THE ENEMY WITHIN

You might find it difficult to cope with the 'slimmer' you. Alison, who dropped from 125 kilograms to 65 kilograms, still regards her body as an 'enemy', which she has done most of her life. 'I have spent so much time obsessed with losing weight and wishing I was physically different,' she says. 'Now it is difficult to like and appreciate the body I hated for so long.'

Changing your perception of yourself can be complicated and difficult. As an adult your body image is entrenched, and altering this image requires a totally different thought process. You are accustomed to unconstructive self-talk about your body – negativity such as 'I look so fat today' – and you

need to develop a more positive image, and you must recognise, accept and enjoy the changes. Initially, feeling and
looking good might be awkward, but eventually it will become
'normal', and your body image will gradually improve.

Are you still avoiding the mirror and wearing shape-
less clothes? It's time to start dressing because you like the
clothes you are buying, not to cover or camouflage your figure.
Attempt activities you would not have participated in before:
go to the gym, wear a swimsuit to the beach. You might feel
self-conscious initially, so ease into these changes – wear a
swimsuit and shorts around the house before wearing them
to the beach, the gym or other public place. Enjoy your new
confidence and healthier body by getting involved in different
physical activities – dance classes, sport, belly dancing or ball-
room dancing. If you still feel self-conscious, remember that
everyone else is too busy worrying about themselves and their
routines to focus on your perceived figure faults!

Remember that your size – whether large or small – is not
the most significant thing about you. Pay attention to other,
more important aspects of your self-image, such as your intel-
ligence, competence and sense of humour. And remember to
keep a balance in your life between family, work, socialising,
exercising, eating and relaxing. Have faith in your ability to
conquer your weight problems forever. I know you can lose
weight and keep it off, because I have achieved it and have
helped so many people to succeed in doing just that!

All you have to do is obey the 10 Commandments of successful weight loss:

1

A LIFESTYLE, NOT A DIET

2

GET ORGANISED

3

EAT SMALL

4

LEARN TO LEAVE FOOD ON YOUR PLATE

5

NEVER FEEL DEPRIVED

6

MAKE A MEAL OF IT

7

EAT SLOWLY

8

ENJOY YOUR FOOD

9

MOVE IT!

10

BALANCE YOUR LIFE

CHAPTER 16

Weekly menus to keep you trim

It is often difficult to plan menus from one day to the next. I do not want you to feel anxious about your meal plan, so to assist you with ideas for meals and snacks I have included a few menus with delicious, easy-to-prepare recipes.

The menus are well-balanced and high in nutrients. They offer variety in tastes and textures – something to satisfy all your senses and desires.

Enjoy!

Dairy and fat requirement
2 cups low-fat milk daily
2 teaspoons fat (butter, oil, margarine, peanut butter or avocado) daily

Exercise requirement
Forty-five minutes of aerobic exercise – walk, swim, gym session – each day. Work out a plan to add a little more exercise to your life every day. Remember, the exercise should be strenuous enough to make you a little breathless and to work up a sweat. If you have any pain or are gasping for breath, you are overdoing

it. Remember, you must consult a doctor before beginning any exercise regime.

Fluid requirement
Water, diet cordial, diet soft drinks, unflavoured mineral water, tea, coffee, herbal teas, cocoa, Bonox/Bovril, 1 cup of tomato juice per day.

Flavour requirement
All foods must be tasty, so be sure to add herbs and spices to your meals, and make use of condiments such as sweet chilli sauce, soy sauce, oyster sauce, tomato sauce, barbecue sauce, mustard, chutney, pickles, pepper, Tabasco and curry paste/powder.

Salads and stir-fries
I have recommended some meals be served with 2 cups salad or 2 cups stir-fried vegetables. The salad and vegetables are from the free foods list (see pages 43–44) – just help yourself to approximately 2 cups from these items. When preparing your salad, use low-joule dressings, lemon juice, cracked black pepper or balsamic vinegar as a dressing. When preparing your vegetables, remember that you can buy stir-fry vegetables at the supermarket, or combine your own choices from the free foods list. You can stir-fry the vegetables in any of the free food list condiments, such as sweet chilli sauce, oyster sauce or soy sauce.

Bread
Choose whichever bread is your favourite (see page 124 for the lowdown on different types of bread and their nutrient content) – remember, each slice of bread is 30 grams. In some cases I have stipulated rye bread or wholegrain, just to add variety, but in all other cases it is up to you.

Exchanges

You can make exchanges using the meal plan guide in Chapter 3 – remember, you can only exchange a carbohydrate for another carbohydrate; and never exchange for a treat more than once a day.

(Meals with recipes are designated by capital letters.)

WEEK 1

Day 1

Breakfast: 1 cup berries with 200 grams low-fat yoghurt

Morning tea: 1 small peach

Lunch: Tuna salad: 100 grams canned tuna, 2 cups mixed salad, 2 slices canned beetroot, 6 olives, with low-fat salad dressing or balsamic vinegar or lemon juice

Afternoon tea: 1 small nectarine

Dinner: WARM PORK, BEAN AND TOMATO SALAD

Supper: 1 small mango or 30 grams (3 squares) chocolate

Day 2

Breakfast: ½ cup high-fibre cereal

Morning tea: 1 plum

Lunch: 30 grams tasty cheese on 2 slices bread (toasted if desired), with salad

Afternoon tea: 1 small nectarine or 2 ORANGE BITES

Dinner: CHICKEN MUSHROOM PASTA

Supper: Low-joule jelly (there's no limit here, but remember to only eat until you are comfortable, never until you are full or bloated)

Day 3

Breakfast: ½ cup high-fibre cereal

Morning tea: 25 grams nuts and raisins

Lunch: Bread roll with rare roast beef, seeded mustard and salad

Afternoon tea: 100 grams Fruche Lite or 30 grams (3 squares) chocolate or 2 ORANGE BITES
Dinner: MARINATED TUNA AND SPINACH SALAD
Supper: 1 icy pole (Calippo, Weiss bar) or 125 grams canned fruit

Day 4

Breakfast: 1 slice sourdough toast with chopped banana and a drizzle of honey
Morning tea: 1 small pear
Lunch: Roast turkey breast sandwich: 2 slices rye bread, 60 grams roast turkey breast, alfalfa sprouts, 2 slices tomato, 2 slices beetroot, grated carrot, shredded lettuce, cranberry jelly
Afternoon tea: 2 crackers with tomato and black pepper or 2 ORANGE BITES
Dinner: VEAL WITH LEMON SAGE CREAM served with 2 cups salad
Supper: 10 cherries

Day 5

Breakfast: 1 poached egg with grilled tomato and mushrooms
Morning tea: 200 grams low-fat yoghurt
Lunch: Greek salad: 60 grams fetta cheese, lettuce, tomato, capsicum, cucumber, red onion, 6 kalamata olives, with low-joule dressing or balsamic vinegar or lemon juice
Afternoon tea: 1 cup cubed watermelon
Dinner: FISH WITH TOMATO DILL SAUCE served with 2 cups salad
Supper: 1 small mango

Day 6

Breakfast: ½ cup high-fibre cereal
Morning tea: 1 plum

Lunch: 1 chicken-and-salad wrap: 1 wrap with 60 grams chicken breast, mustard or pickles and salad
Afternoon tea: 1 apricot
Dinner: SPICY COUSCOUS
Supper: 10 cherries or 30 grams (3 squares) chocolate or 1 icy pole

Day 7
Breakfast: 1 slice toast with 1 teaspoon peanut butter or jam or honey
Morning tea: 1 small peach
Lunch: Miso soup, 2 sushi rolls
Afternoon tea: 1 small nectarine or 2 ORANGE BITES
Dinner: CREAMY LAMB BAKES served with 2 cups stir-fried vegetables
Supper: Low-joule jelly

Recipes for Week 1

WARM PORK, BEAN AND TOMATO SALAD

<u>SERVES 4</u>

400 g sweet potatoes, peeled and cut into 2-cm thick slices
1 teaspoon olive oil
400 g pork fillet
2 medium tomatoes, seeded and cut into wedges
300 g can butter beans, drained and rinsed
4 spring onions, thinly sliced
½ cup coarsely chopped fresh parsley
⅓ cup no-fat French dressing
1 teaspoon finely grated lemon rind
salt and pepper, to taste

Bring a large saucepan of water to the boil. Add sweet potatoes and cook, uncovered, for 6 minutes or until just tender. Remove saucepan from heat, rinse under cold water and then drain sweet potatoes well and set aside.

Add oil to a heated non-stick frying pan. Add pork and cook, turning frequently, for 12–15 minutes or until tender but still slightly pink in the centre. Remove pork from frying pan and leave to rest for 5 minutes, then cut into thin slices.

As pork is resting, return frying pan to heat, add sweet potatoes and cook until browned on both sides and heated through.

In a large bowl, combine sweet potatoes, tomatoes, beans, spring onions and parsley. Add pork, then drizzle combined dressing and lemon rind over, season with salt and pepper and serve.

CHICKEN MUSHROOM PASTA

<u>SERVES 4</u>

6 thin low-fat chicken sausages
2 teaspoons vegetable oil
200 g button mushrooms, sliced
2 cloves garlic, crushed
425 g can crushed tomatoes, undrained
salt and pepper, to taste
1 cup elbow pasta (or your favourite pasta)
150 g broccoli florets
½ cup fresh basil leaves, shredded

Add sausages to a saucepan of cold water, then place the pan over heat and bring water to the boil. Reduce heat and simmer for 5 minutes, then remove saucepan from heat and drain sausages. Cut sausages diagonally into 3-cm pieces and set aside.

Heat oil in a large saucepan. Add mushrooms and garlic, and cook, stirring, until mushrooms are soft. Add tomatoes, increase heat and bring to the boil, then reduce heat and simmer, uncovered, for 5 minutes before seasoning with salt and pepper.

Meanwhile, bring a large saucepan of water to the boil. Add pasta and cook, uncovered, until just tender. Add broccoli and cook for 1 minute, then remove saucepan from heat. Drain pasta and broccoli well and then return to pan.

Add tomato mixture, basil and sausages to pasta, and toss gently to combine before serving.

MARINATED TUNA AND SPINACH SALAD
SERVES 4

100 g baby spinach leaves
1 medium carrot, grated
½ red capsicum, thinly sliced
4 spring onions, thinly sliced
2 tablespoons light soy sauce
1 teaspoon sesame oil
2 teaspoons white wine vinegar
2 teaspoons caster sugar
2 teaspoons toasted sesame seeds
600 g tuna steak
⅓ cup teriyaki sauce
cooking oil spray

In a large bowl, combine spinach with carrot, capsicum and spring onions. In a jug, combine soy sauce, sesame oil, white wine vinegar, caster sugar and sesame seeds. Mix well and then pour over spinach mixture. Toss well and set salad aside.

Place tuna in a large bowl and pour over the teriyaki sauce. Cover and refrigerate for 30 minutes.

Drain tuna. Spray a heated grill plate with oil. Add tuna and cook on both sides until lightly browned and cooked to your liking (1–2 minutes for rare, 2–4 minutes for well done). Remove from heat, cover and set aside to rest for a few minutes before cutting into thick slices.

Arrange salad on serving plates, then top with tuna and serve.

VEAL WITH LEMON SAGE CREAM
SERVES 4

¼ cup reduced-fat mayonnaise
1 tablespoon light sour cream
½ clove garlic, crushed
1 teaspoon Dijon mustard
½ teaspoon finely grated lemon rind
1 tablespoon lemon juice
2 teaspoons finely chopped fresh sage
salt and pepper, to taste
2 teaspoons olive oil
500 g veal steaks
½ teaspoon lemon pepper seasoning

In a small jug, combine mayonnaise, sour cream, garlic, mustard, lemon rind, lemon juice and sage, and season with salt and pepper. Cover and refrigerate until ready to serve.

Heat oil in a non-stick frying pan. Sprinkle veal with lemon pepper seasoning on both sides and cook for 2 minutes on each side or until browned and tender.

Arrange veal on serving plates. Spread lemon sage cream over veal and serve with 2 cups salad.

FISH WITH TOMATO DILL SAUCE
SERVES 4

cooking oil spray

4 × 150 g thin fish fillets

1 tablespoon finely grated Parmesan cheese

cooking oil spray

1 small onion, finely chopped

1 clove garlic, crushed

400 g can chopped tomatoes

½ cup vegetable stock

2 tablespoons chopped fresh dill

2 teaspoons baby capers

salt and pepper, to taste

Spray oil over both sides of fish and place fish on an oven tray. Sprinkle cheese over fish and cook under a hot grill, without turning, until browned and cooked through.

As fish is cooking, spray a heated saucepan with oil. Add onion and garlic, and cook, stirring, for 2–3 minutes or until soft. Add tomatoes and stock, and bring to the boil, then reduce heat and simmer, uncovered, for 10 minutes or until the sauce has thickened. Stir in dill and capers, and season with salt and pepper.

Arrange fish on serving plates and pour tomato dill sauce over. Serve with 2 cups salad.

SPICY COUSCOUS

SERVES 4

1 tablespoon chopped fresh parsley
1 tablespoon chopped fresh mint
½ cup plain skim-milk yoghurt
cooking oil spray
2 medium onions, thinly sliced
1 clove garlic, crushed
2 teaspoons hot curry paste
1 zucchini, thinly sliced
1½ cups chicken stock
½ cup frozen peas
1½ cups plain couscous
2 tomatoes, chopped
salt and pepper, to taste

In a bowl, combine herbs and yoghurt, and set aside.

Spray a heated non-stick frying pan with oil. Add onions and garlic, and cook, stirring, for 2–3 minutes or until onions are soft and translucent. Stir in curry paste and cook for 30 seconds, then add zucchini and cook, stirring, for 1 minute.

Add stock and peas, then increase heat and bring to the boil. Remove from heat and stir in couscous, then leave to rest, covered, for 5 minutes. Using a fork, gently stir in tomatoes. Season with salt and pepper.

Arrange couscous on serving plates, drizzle yoghurt over and serve.

CREAMY LAMB BAKES

<u>SERVES 4</u>

400 g lean minced lamb

1 clove garlic, crushed

400 g can crushed tomatoes, undrained

½ cup vegetable stock

1 tablespoon tomato paste

¼ cup chopped fresh basil

salt and pepper, to taste

2 tablespoons plain flour

2 cups skim milk

⅓ cup finely grated Parmesan cheese

Preheat oven to 190°C.

Heat a non-stick frying pan. Add lamb in batches (cooking in batches will brown the meat rather than stew it) and cook, stirring occasionally, until browned and cooked through. Return all lamb to pan and add garlic, tomatoes, stock and tomato paste. Increase heat and bring to the boil, then reduce heat and simmer, uncovered, for 15 minutes or until liquid has slightly thickened. Stir in basil, and season with salt and pepper. Remove from heat.

In a small saucepan, blend flour with ¼ cup of the skim milk until smooth. Place saucepan over heat and stir in remaining milk. Continue stirring until sauce boils and thickens, then stir in 1 tablespoon of the cheese.

Divide lamb mixture among four shallow individual ovenproof dishes. Top with cheese sauce and sprinkle with remaining cheese. Bake, uncovered, for 20 minutes or until lightly browned. Serve with 2 cups stir-fried vegetables.

ORANGE BITES

MARKS 70 BITES

185 g butter
2 teaspoons grated orange rind
⅓ cup icing sugar
1½ cups plain flour
5 tablespoons custard powder

Preheat oven to 180°C. Line oven trays with baking paper.

In a small bowl, combine butter, orange rind and icing sugar. With an electric mixer, mix until light and fluffy.

In a separate bowl, sift flour and custard powder. Add flour mix to butter mix and stir with a wooden spoon to combine.

Roll rounded teaspoons of mixture into small balls and place about 3 cm apart on oven trays. With a fork, press down lightly on each ball to flatten slightly.

Bake for 12 minutes or until lightly browned. Cool biscuits on trays and then store in an airtight container. (Leftover bites can be stored in an airtight container in the freezer for up to 3 months.)

WEEK 2

Day 1

Breakfast: 1 grapefruit and 1 boiled egg

Morning tea: 1 small peach or 1 small apple

Lunch: Chicken salad: 120 grams chicken breast (grilled and shredded), 2 cups mixed salad, 2 slices canned beetroot, 6 olives, with low-fat dressing or balsamic vinegar

Afternoon tea: 1 small nectarine or 1 small pear

Dinner: LAMB WITH BEAN SALAD

Supper: 200 grams low-fat yoghurt or 30 grams (3 squares) chocolate

Day 2

Breakfast: 1 slice toast with grilled tomato and mushrooms and black pepper

Morning tea: 1 apricot or 1 kiwifruit

Lunch: Cottage cheese sandwich: 2 slices bread with 90 grams low-fat cottage cheese and salad

Afternoon tea: 1 plum or 2 BUTTERY COOKIES

Dinner: TOMATO, ROCKET AND SALMON SALAD

Supper: 125 grams canned fruit

Day 3

Breakfast: ½ cup high-fibre cereal

Morning tea: 25 grams nuts and raisins

Lunch: Bread roll with 100 grams tuna and salad

Afternoon tea: 100 grams Fruche Lite or 30 grams (3 squares) chocolate or 2 BUTTERY COOKIES

Dinner: CHILLI PORK served with 2 cups stir-fried vegetables

Supper: 1 icy pole (Calippo, Weiss bar) or 125 grams canned fruit

Day 4
Breakfast: 1 slice sourdough toast with 45 grams ricotta and a drizzle of honey
Morning tea: 1 small apple
Lunch: Rare roast beef sandwich: 2 slices wholegrain bread, 50 grams rare roast beef, alfalfa sprouts, 2 slices tomato, 2 slices beetroot, grated carrot, shredded lettuce, mustard
Afternoon tea: 2 crackers with tomato and black pepper or 2 BUTTERY COOKIES
Dinner: CHICKEN CHICKPEA SALAD
Supper: 10 cherries

Day 5
Breakfast: ½ cup high-fibre cereal
Morning tea: 200 grams low-fat yoghurt
Lunch: Cheese-and-salad sandwich: 2 slices wholegrain bread, 30 grams cheddar cheese and salad
Afternoon tea: 1 cup cubed rockmelon
Dinner: WARM BEEF WITH POTATOES
Supper: 1 small mango

Day 6
Breakfast: 1 poached egg on toast with grilled tomato and mushrooms
Morning tea: 1 plum
Lunch: 1 chicken-and-salad wrap: 1 wrap with 60 grams chicken breast and salad
Afternoon tea: 1 apricot
Dinner: FRIED RICE
Supper: 10 cherries or 30 grams (3 squares) chocolate or 1 icy pole

Day 7

Breakfast: ½ cup high-fibre cereal

Morning tea: 2 plain biscuits or 2 crackers with jam or Vegemite or honey

Lunch: Miso soup, 2 sushi rolls

Afternoon tea: 1 small mango or 2 BUTTERY COOKIES

Dinner: HONEY SOY CHICKEN SALAD

Supper: Low-joule jelly

Recipes for Week 2

LAMB WITH BEAN SALAD
<u>SERVES 4</u>

1 red capsicum, chopped
100 g mixed lettuce leaves
200 g green beans, chopped
⅓ cup light mayonnaise
1 teaspoon wholegrain mustard
1 teaspoon honey
1 tablespoon chopped fresh mint leaves
1 tablespoon chopped fresh parsley
1 tablespoon lemon juice
salt and pepper, to taste
cooking oil spray
8 lamb cutlets

In a large bowl, combine capsicum and lettuce leaves.

Bring a medium saucepan of water to the boil. Add beans and cook for 5 minutes or until just tender, then remove from heat and drain. Rinse beans under cold water and then add to capsicum and lettuce leaves.

In a jug, combine mayonnaise, mustard and honey. Mix well and then pour over salad. Toss well.

In a small bowl, combine herbs and lemon juice, then season with salt and pepper.

Spray a heated grill plate with oil. Add lamb cutlets and cook for 3 minutes on each side or until browned and cooked through. Remove from heat and arrange on plates. Sprinkle herbs over cutlets, and serve with bean salad.

TOMATO, ROCKET AND SALMON SALAD

<u>SERVES 4</u>

4 large Roma tomatoes, quartered lengthways
sea salt and cracked black pepper, to taste
2 tablespoons grated Parmesan cheese
150 g rocket leaves, trimmed and torn
1 small red onion, thinly sliced
2 × 210 g cans pink salmon, drained
¼ cup fat-free lemon-lime-and-cracked-pepper dressing

Preheat oven to 120°C.

Place tomatoes skin-side down on an oven tray and sprinkle with salt and pepper. Cook for 1 hour, or until soft, then remove from oven and set aside to cool.

In a large bowl, combine cooled tomatoes, cheese, rocket leaves and onion. Add flaked salmon and drizzle with dressing. Toss gently before serving.

CHILLI PORK

<u>SERVES 4</u>

1 tablespoon brown sugar
1 tablespoon sweet chilli sauce
1 tablespoon lime juice
2 teaspoons grated fresh ginger
1 clove garlic, crushed
½ teaspoon five spice powder
4 × 125 g pork leg steaks
cooking oil spray

In a large bowl, combine sugar, sweet chilli sauce, lime juice, ginger, garlic and five spice powder. Add pork and mix well to thoroughly coat pork with marinade. Cover and refrigerate for 15 minutes.

Remove pork from refrigerator and drain, reserving marinade in a bowl. Spray a heated grill plate with oil. Add pork and cook, brushing with remaining marinade and turning frequently, for 10 minutes or until browned and tender on both sides. Arrange pork on serving plates and serve with 2 cups stir-fried vegetables.

CHICKEN CHICKPEA SALAD

<u>SERVES 4</u>

400 g chicken tenderloins
2 teaspoons Cajun seasoning
1 clove garlic, crushed
300 g can chickpeas, rinsed and drained
1 small red onion, finely chopped
1 cup coarsely chopped fresh parsley
1 Lebanese cucumber, finely chopped
100 g button mushrooms, thinly sliced
2 tablespoons lemon juice
2 tablespoons no-fat French dressing
salt and pepper, to taste
cooking oil spray

In a large bowl, combine chicken, seasoning and garlic. Mix well, cover and refrigerate for 30 minutes.

In a large bowl, combine chickpeas, onion, parsley, cucumber, mushrooms, lemon juice and dressing. Season with salt and pepper and toss well.

Remove chicken from fridge. Spray a heated non-stick frying pan with oil. Add chicken and cook, turning frequently, for 10 minutes or until browned on both sides and cooked through. Remove from heat and slice. Arrange salad on serving plates, place chicken on top and serve.

WARM BEEF WITH POTATOES

<u>SERVES 4</u>

⅓ cup light sour cream

1 tablespoon wholegrain mustard

1 cup fresh basil leaves, firmly packed

2 cloves garlic, peeled

1 tablespoon lemon juice

salt and pepper, to taste

100 g baby spinach

1 tablespoon pine nuts, toasted

200 g baby chat potatoes

500 g rump steak, fat trimmed

2 teaspoons olive oil

In the bowl of a food processor, combine sour cream, mustard, basil leaves, garlic and lemon juice, and season with salt and pepper. Process for 30 minutes, then turn off motor and scrape down the sides. Process for a further 30 seconds or until pureed.

In a salad bowl, combine spinach and pine nuts, and set aside.

Bring a large saucepan of salted water to the boil. Add potatoes and cook, uncovered, for 15 minutes or until just tender. Remove saucepan from heat and drain potatoes. Cut into thick slices and set aside.

Heat a non-stick frying pan. Add beef and cook for 3 minutes on each side or until browned and tender. Transfer beef to a plate, then cover and leave to rest for 5 minutes. Thinly slice beef, add to salad bowl and combine.

Drain the frying pan, then return to heat and add oil. Add potato slices in a single layer. Cook for 2–3 minutes or until lightly browned. Add potatoes and salad dressing to salad bowl, toss well and serve.

FRIED RICE

<u>SERVES 4</u>

1 cup white long grain rice

2 zucchini, thinly sliced

2 teaspoons vegetable oil

2 eggs, lightly beaten

1 clove garlic, crushed

1 teaspoon finely grated fresh ginger

1 tablespoon mild curry paste

4 spring onions, sliced

1 stick celery, sliced

2 tablespoons teriyaki sauce

Line an oven tray with absorbent paper. Bring a large pan of salted water to the boil. Add rice and cook, uncovered, for 10 minutes or until tender. Remove from heat and drain. Rinse rice under cold water and drain well. Spread rice over absorbent paper to dry completely.

Bring a medium saucepan of water to the boil. Add zucchini and cook for 3 minutes or until just tender. Remove from heat and drain, then rinse zucchini under cold water and drain again.

In a wok or large non-stick frying pan, heat half the oil. Pour in eggs and swirl wok or pan to make a thin omelette. Cook for 1–2 minutes or until set, then remove from pan. Roll up omelette tightly as if it were a pancake, and thinly slice.

Heat remaining oil in the wok. Add garlic, ginger, curry paste and spring onions, and stir-fry for 1 minute. Add celery, rice, and teriyaki sauce, and stir-fry for 2 minutes or until rice is heated through. Add omelette slices, and stir-fry until combined.

HONEY SOY CHICKEN SALAD

SERVES 4

2 tablespoons soy sauce

⅓ cup honey

1 clove garlic, crushed

4 fresh red Thai chillies, seeded and finely chopped

600 g chicken breast fillets, thinly sliced

300 g snow peas

1 tablespoon peanut oil

1 small carrot, sliced into ribbons

2 cups Savoy cabbage, finely shredded

1 medium red capsicum, thinly sliced

1 medium yellow capsicum, thinly sliced

4 spring onions, thinly sliced

½ cup fresh mint leaves

2 tablespoons lime juice

2 teaspoons sesame seed oil

In a medium bowl, combine soy sauce, honey, garlic and half of the chilli. Add chicken and toss to thoroughly coat chicken in chilli mixture. Cover and refrigerate (for at least 15 minutes) until required.

Bring a medium saucepan of water to the boil. Add snow peas and cook for 1 minute until just tender. Remove from heat and drain, then immediately rinse under cold water and drain again. Transfer to a salad bowl.

Remove chicken from refrigerator and drain. In a wok or large non-stick frying pan, heat peanut oil. Add chicken in batches and cook, turning frequently, for 3 minutes or until browned and cooked through.

Add chicken to the salad bowl, and then add carrot, cabbage, capsicum, spring onion, mint leaves, lime juice, sesame seed oil and remaining chilli. Toss gently to combine and serve.

BUTTERY COOKIES
MAKES 70 COOKIES

2 cups plain flour
½ cup self-raising flour
250 g butter, softened
1 teaspoon aniseed extract
½ cup caster sugar
1 egg yolk

In a bowl, combine plain flour and self-raising flour, and set aside.

In a large bowl, combine butter, aniseed extract, caster sugar and egg yolk. With an electric mixer, mix until smooth and creamy. With a wooden spoon, stir in flours in two batches, until you have a soft dough.

Transfer mixture to a smooth, clean benchtop. Divide mixture in half and roll each half into a log shape about 3 cm in diameter. Wrap each log in plastic wrap and refrigerate for 1 hour.

Preheat oven to 180°C. Line oven trays with baking paper.

Transfer logs to your benchtop. With a sharp knife, cut each log into 3 mm slices and place on oven trays. Cook for 8 minutes or until lightly browned. Remove biscuits from oven and leave to rest on tray for 5 minutes, before transferring to wire racks to cool. Store in an airtight container. (Leftover cookies can be stored in an airtight container in the freezer for up to 3 months.)

WEEK 3

Day 1

Breakfast: 2 passionfruit with 100 grams Fruche Lite

Morning tea: 1 small nectarine or 1 small orange

Lunch: Fetta cheese salad: 60 grams fetta cheese, 2 cups salad vegetables, 2 slices canned beetroot, 6 olives, with low-joule dressing or balsamic vinegar

Afternoon tea: 1 mango or 1 small banana

Dinner: SAFFRON VEGETABLE RICE

Supper: Low-joule jelly

Day 2

Breakfast: 1 poached egg with grilled tomato and mushrooms and black pepper

Morning tea: 1 small peach or 2 fresh figs

Lunch: Tuna-and-salad sandwich: 2 slices bread with 100 grams tuna and salad

Afternoon tea: 1 small apple or 2 ORANGE BISCUITS

Dinner: CHICKEN BEAN SALAD

Supper: 1 apricot or 2 passionfruit

Day 3

Breakfast: ½ cup high-fibre cereal

Morning tea: 1 plum

Lunch: Bread roll with 90 grams cottage cheese and salad

Afternoon tea: 1 low-fat yoghurt or 25 grams (3 squares) chocolate or 2 ORANGE BISCUITS

Dinner: STEAK WITH CREAMY POTATO SALAD

Supper: 1 icy pole (Calippo, Weiss bar) or 125 grams canned fruit

Day 4
Breakfast: 1 slice sourdough toast with small banana and a drizzle of honey
Morning tea: 1 small peach
Lunch: Roast turkey breast sandwich: 2 slices rye bread, 60 grams roast turkey breast, alfalfa sprouts, 2 slices tomato, 2 slices canned beetroot, grated carrot, shredded lettuce, cranberry jelly
Afternoon tea: 2 crackers with tomato and black pepper or 2 ORANGE BISCUITS
Dinner: SPICY LAMB STIR-FRY
Supper: 10 cherries

Day 5
Breakfast: ½ cup high-fibre cereal
Morning tea: 200 grams low-fat yoghurt
Lunch: Chicken-and-salad sandwich: 2 slices wholegrain bread, 120 grams chicken breast, flavoured with pickles or mustard
Afternoon tea: 1 small mango
Dinner: MEDITERRANEAN FISH
Supper: 1 cup cubed watermelon

Day 6
Breakfast: 1 cup berries with 1 chopped banana
Morning tea: 2 crackers with a thin spread of jam, honey or Vegemite
Lunch: Cheese-and-salad wrap: 1 wrap with 30 grams grated cheese and salad (toast if desired)
Afternoon tea: 1 apricot
Dinner: CHINESE-STYLE PORK served with 2 cups salad
Supper: 1 cup cubed honeydew melon

Day 7
Breakfast: 1 slice toast with 1 scrambled egg and tomato
Morning tea: 1 plum
Lunch: Miso soup, 2 sushi rolls
Afternoon tea: 1 small mango or 2 ORANGE BISCUITS
Dinner: CHICKEN AND CABBAGE SALAD
Supper: Low-joule jelly

Recipes for Week 3

SAFFRON VEGETABLE RICE
SERVES 4

cooking oil spray
1 onion, chopped
1 clove garlic, crushed
½ teaspoon saffron powder
2 medium zucchini, thinly sliced
2 carrots, chopped
½ cup frozen corn kernels
1 cup long grain rice
2 cups vegetable stock
¼ cup coarsely chopped fresh parsley
salt and pepper, to taste

Spray a heated non-stick frying pan with oil. Add onion and garlic, and cook, stirring, for 2–3 minutes or until soft. Add saffron powder, zucchini, carrots, corn and rice, and cook, stirring, for 1 minute.

Add stock, then increase heat and bring mixture to the boil. Reduce heat and simmer, covered, for 15–20 minutes or until liquid is absorbed and rice is tender. Stir in parsley, season with salt and pepper and serve.

CHICKEN BEAN SALAD

<u>SERVES 4</u>

¼ cup no-fat plain yoghurt
¼ cup 98% fat-free mayonnaise
1 clove garlic, crushed
2 teaspoons Dijon mustard
salt and pepper, to taste
1 bunch (6 spears) asparagus, cut into 2-cm lengths
200 g green beans, halved crossways
½ cup frozen peas
500 g chicken tenderloins
1 red capsicum, thinly sliced
300 g can butter beans, rinsed and drained

In a jug, combine yoghurt, mayonnaise, garlic and mustard, and season with salt and pepper. Whisk well and set aside.

Bring a large saucepan of water to the boil. Add asparagus and boil for 2–5 minutes, depending on thickness. Using a slotted spoon, remove asparagus from water (leave water boiling) and plunge into a large bowl of iced water. Remove asparagus (keeping iced water in bowl), drain well and transfer to a salad bowl. Add beans and peas to the same saucepan of boiling water and boil for 3–4 minutes or until tender. Remove pan from heat and drain over a sieve. Place sieve in the bowl of iced water and leave to rest for 1 minute. Drain greens and add to salad bowl. Combine greens and set aside.

Heat an oiled grill plate. Add chicken and cook for 3 minutes on each side or until browned and tender. Remove from heat, cover and leave to rest for 5 minutes.

Slice chicken into strips and add to the salad bowl. Add capsicum, butter beans and then dressing, mix well and serve.

STEAK WITH CREAMY POTATO SALAD
SERVES 4

410 g can potatoes, drained and cut into thick slices
250 g punnet cherry tomatoes, halved
100 g baby spinach leaves
2 spring onions, finely sliced
½ cup 99% fat-free Dijonnaise
1 tablespoon fat-free French dressing
2 tablespoons chopped fresh chives
4 × 125 g fillet steaks
cooking oil spray
salt and pepper, to taste

In a jug, combine Dijonnaise and French dressing.

In a large bowl, combine potatoes, tomatoes, spinach, spring onions and combined dressing. Toss through chives.

Lightly spray a heated grill plate with oil. Add steaks and cook on both sides until browned and cooked to your liking (2–3 minutes for rare, 3–5 minutes for well done). Season with salt and pepper.

Serve steaks with creamy potato salad.

SPICY LAMB STIR-FRY

<u>SERVES 4</u>

1 tablespoon sweet chilli sauce

2 tablespoons soy sauce

1 tablespoon oyster sauce

2 cloves garlic, crushed

1 teaspoon sweet paprika

500 g lamb strips

1 teaspoon sesame oil

1 onion, cut into wedges

2 carrots, thinly sliced

250 g broccoli florets

1 red capsicum, sliced

In a large jug, combine sweet chilli sauce, soy sauce, oyster sauce, garlic and paprika. Mix well. Place lamb in a bowl and pour over half the marinade, setting remaining marinade aside in the jug. Leave lamb to rest for 15 minutes.

Heat oil in a large wok or non-stick frying pan. Add lamb in batches (cooking in batches will brown the meat rather than stew it) and stir-fry for 2 minutes or until tender. Remove lamb from wok and set aside on a plate as you stir-fry the remaining lamb. Place remaining lamb on plate and leave wok over heat.

Add onion and carrots to wok, and stir-fry for 2 minutes or until carrots are soft. Add broccoli and capsicum, and stir-fry for 2 minutes or until broccoli is tender. Return lamb to wok and pour over remaining marinade. Stir-fry for 1 minute or until heated through, then serve.

MEDITERRANEAN FISH

SERVES 4

1 red capsicum
1 onion, sliced
1 clove garlic, crushed
2 medium tomatoes, chopped
2 teaspoons drained baby capers
¼ cup tomato juice
1 tablespoon sundried tomato pesto
salt and pepper, to taste
cooking oil spray
4 × 150 g fish fillets

Cut capsicum into quarters, then remove seeds and membranes. Place capsicum skin-side up on an oven tray and place under grill. Cook until skin blisters and blackens, then remove from heat. Peel skin from capsicum and then cut capsicum into thin strips.

In a small frying pan, combine capsicum, onion, garlic, tomatoes, capers, tomato juice and pesto. Stir over heat for 2 minutes or until warmed through and season with salt and pepper.

As vegetables are cooking, spray a heated non-stick frying pan with oil. Add fish and cook for 2–3 minutes in each side or until lightly browned and tender.

Arrange vegetables on serving plates, place fish on top and serve.

CHINESE-STYLE PORK
SERVES 4

1 tablespoon honey
1 teaspoon Chinese barbecue sauce
1 tablespoon dark soy sauce
4 × 125 g pork steaks, fat trimmed
2 corn cobs, husks removed
cooking oil spray
salt and pepper, to taste

In a large bowl, combine honey and sauces. Add pork and mix well to thoroughly coat pork with marinade.

Cut corn cobs into four equal rounds. Spray lightly with oil, and season with salt and pepper.

Heat an oiled grill plate or barbecue hot plate. Add pork and corn. Cook pork for 3 minutes on each side or until browned all over and slightly pink in the centre. Turn corn frequently for 2 minutes on each side to brown.

Serve pork and corn with 2 cups salad.

CHICKEN AND CABBAGE SALAD

SERVES 4

1 large whole barbecued chicken

4 cups Chinese cabbage, finely shredded

4 spring onions, thinly sliced

½ cup finely chopped fresh basil, firmly packed

2 cloves garlic, crushed

2 tablespoons sweet chilli sauce

2 tablespoons lime juice

2 tablespoons fish sauce

2 tablespoons water

1 tablespoon sugar

Remove skin and bones from the chicken. Using your fingers, tear meat into shreds. In a large bowl, combine chicken, cabbage, spring onion and basil. Mix by hand to thoroughly combine.

In a jar with a screw-top lid, combine garlic, sweet chilli sauce, lime juice, fish sauce, water and sugar. Tighten lid and shake jar well, then drizzle dressing over chicken salad. Toss gently to combine and serve.

ORANGE BISCUITS

<u>MAKES 50 BISCUITS</u>

125 g butter, at room temperature
60 g cream cheese, at room temperature
2 teaspoons grated orange rind
1 teaspoon grated lemon rind
1 cup caster sugar
1 egg
2 cups plain flour, sifted

Preheat oven to 180°C. Line oven trays with baking paper.

In a large bowl, combine butter, cream cheese, rinds and caster sugar. With an electric mixer, mix until smooth. Add egg and continue beating until just combined. Stir in sifted flour and mix until a soft dough forms. Divide mixture into two portions, wrap each portion in plastic wrap, cover and refrigerate for 1 hour.

Roll each portion between two sheets of baking paper to 4-mm thickness. (Rolling the dough between the sheets of baking paper will stop it sticking to your benchtop and creating the need to add extra flour, which will change the consistency of the biscuits.) Using a 6.5-cm biscuit cutter (this gives you the correct amount of kilojoules per biscuit), cut out rounds. Place about 5 cm apart on oven trays and bake for 15 minutes or until lightly browned. Remove from oven and leave on trays for 5 minutes before transferring to wire racks to cool. Store biscuits in an airtight container. (Leftover biscuits can be stored in an airtight container in the freezer for up to 3 months.)

WEEK 4

Day 1

Breakfast: 3 passionfruit with 200 grams low-fat yoghurt

Morning tea: 1 small nectarine

Lunch: Pastrami sandwich: 2 slices rye bread, 50 grams pastrami with fat trimmed off, seeded mustard, shredded lettuce, tomato, 2 slices canned beetroot, grated carrot, cucumber, ½ tablespoon fresh parsley leaves, mustard

Afternoon tea: 1 small nectarine

Dinner: GARLIC AND LEMON VEAL with 2 cups salad

Supper: 1 small orange

Day 2

Breakfast: 1 poached egg with grilled tomato and mushrooms

Morning tea: 1 slice raisin toast and jam

Lunch: Chicken salad: 120 grams chicken, 1 cup lettuce, 2 tomatoes (quartered), 4 slices canned beetroot, few slices red onion, ½ cup grated carrot, few slices cucumber, 2 radishes, few slices capsicum, with low-fat salad dressing

Afternoon tea: 1 small apple

Dinner: FISH IN OYSTER SAUCE with 3 serves steamed or stir-fried vegetables

Supper: 30 grams (3 squares) chocolate or 2 SULTANA BISCUITS or 10 cherries

Day 3

Breakfast: ½ cup high-fibre cereal

Morning tea: 1 apricot

Lunch: Tuna salad: 100 grams canned tuna in brine or spring water, 1 cup lettuce, 2 tomatoes (quartered), 4 slices canned beetroot, 1 tablespoon toasted pine nuts, few slices red onion, ½ cup grated carrot, few slices cucumber, 2 radishes, few slices capsicum, with low-fat salad dressing

Afternoon tea: 1 small pear

Dinner: BEEF SKEWERS with 2 serves of vegetables or 2 cups salad

Supper: 1 icy pole (Calippo, Weiss bar) or 1 plum

Day 4

Breakfast: 1 slice wholegrain toast with 1 teaspoon jam or honey or maple syrup

Morning tea: 1 small banana

Lunch: Ricotta cheese sandwich: 2 slices pumpernickel bread, 60 grams ricotta cheese, alfalfa sprouts, 2 slices tomato, 2 slices canned beetroot, grated carrot, shredded lettuce

Afternoon tea: 2 crackers with tomato and black pepper or 2 SULTANA BISCUITS

Dinner: CURRIED POTATO FRITTATA served with 2 cups salad

Supper: 1 small mango

Day 5

Breakfast: 1 cup high-fibre cereal

Morning tea: 1 small peach

Lunch: Small bread roll with roast beef and salad, flavoured with pickles or mustard

Afternoon tea: 1 cup cubed watermelon

Dinner: ORIENTAL PORK SALAD

Supper: 1 cup mixed berries

Day 6

Breakfast: 1 slice toast with 1 teaspoon peanut butter or jam or honey or Vegemite

Morning tea: 25 grams (3 squares) chocolate
Lunch: 1 chicken-mayonnaise-and-salad sandwich: 2 slices
wholegrain bread, 60 grams chicken, 2 teaspoons low-fat mayonnaise
Afternoon tea: 1 apricot
Dinner: CHAR-GRILLED TUNA WITH ROCKET CHICKPEA
SALAD
Supper: 1 cup cubed rockmelon

Day 7
Breakfast: 1 slice toast with scrambled egg and tomato
Morning tea: 1 small peach
Lunch: Miso soup, 2 sushi rolls
Afternoon tea: 1 mango
Dinner: PASTA WITH FRESH TOMATO SAUCE
Supper: Low-joule jelly

Recipes for Week 4

GARLIC AND LEMON VEAL

SERVES 4

2 cloves garlic, crushed
½ cup lemon juice
2 teaspoons lemon herb seasoning
1 teaspoon dried oregano leaves
1 tablespoon Dijon mustard
4 × 125 g veal steaks
⅓ cup water
cooking oil spray

In a large bowl, combine garlic, lemon juice, lemon herb seasoning, oregano leaves and mustard. Whisk until combined, then add veal and mix well to thoroughly coat veal in marinade. Cover and refrigerate for 30 minutes.

Remove veal from refrigerator and drain, reserving marinade in a bowl. Stir water into marinade.

Spray a heated non-stick frying pan with oil. Add veal and cook for 2 minutes on each side or until browned and tender. Transfer veal to a plate and cover with a lid to keep warm. Add marinade mixture to frying pan, then increase heat and stir for 2 minutes or until syrupy.

Drizzle marinade mixture over veal and serve with 2 cups salad.

FISH IN OYSTER SAUCE

SERVES 4

2 teaspoons vegetable oil

2 cloves garlic, crushed

1 tablespoon grated fresh ginger

600 g boneless fish fillets, cut into 1-cm thick slices

3 spring onions, chopped

1 red capsicum, cut into thin strips

1 teaspoon sweet chilli sauce

2 tablespoons oyster sauce

2 tablespoons light soy sauce

1 tablespoon dry sherry

100 g snow peas, trimmed

In a wok or non-stick frying pan, heat half the oil. Add garlic and ginger, and stir-fry for 30 seconds. Add half the fish and cook gently for 2 minutes or until just tender. Leaving the garlic and ginger in the pan, transfer the fish to a plate, and repeat process with remaining oil and fish, then remove fish.

Add spring onions and capsicum to wok, and stir-fry for 2 minutes. Add sauces, sherry and snow peas, and stir-fry for 1 minute.

Return fish to wok, and stir gently for 1 minute or until heated through. Arrange fish on serving plates and pour over sauce. Serve with 3 serves of steamed or stir-fried vegetables.

BEEF SKEWERS

<u>SERVES 4</u>

2 cloves garlic, crushed

½ teaspoon ground coriander

½ teaspoon curry powder

1 tablespoon brown sugar

2 teaspoons sambal oelek (chilli paste)

1 tablespoon fish sauce

500 g lean rump steak, cut into thin strips

1 small carrot, finely chopped

½ Lebanese cucumber, finely chopped

1½ tablespoons white vinegar

¼ cup sugar

1 tablespoon water

In a large bowl, combine garlic, coriander, curry powder, sugar, sambal oelek and fish sauce. Add steak and mix well to thoroughly coat steak, then cover and refrigerate for 30 minutes.

In a bowl, combine carrot and cucumber. Set aside.

In a small saucepan, combine vinegar, sugar and water. Stir over heat until sugar is dissolved, then bring to the boil and cook, uncovered, for 1 minute. Pour hot syrup over carrot and cucumber, and allow to cool.

While sauce is cooling, thread steak onto 8 skewers. Heat a grill plate or barbecue hot plate, and cook skewers, turning frequently, until browned and cooked to your liking (3 minutes each side for medium, 4–5 minutes each side for well done).

Arrange skewers on serving plates and pour carrot–cucumber sauce over the top. Serve with 2 serves of vegetables or 2 cups salad.

CURRIED POTATO FRITTATA

SERVES 4

4 medium (600 g) potatoes
1 teaspoon olive oil
2 teaspoons curry powder
1 red onion, finely chopped
4 eggs, lightly beaten
salt and pepper, to taste
2 tablespoons chopped fresh parsley
3 teaspoons butter, melted

Boil or microwave potatoes until just soft, then allow to cool, and grate into a bowl.

Heat oil in a frying pan. Add curry powder and onion, and cook for 3 minutes or until onion is soft and translucent. Add onion mixture to potatoes, then add eggs, season with salt and pepper and stir in parsley.

Melt butter in a 23-cm frying pan. Add potato mixture and cook over medium heat for 5 minutes, or until well browned underneath and beginning to set. Remove frying pan from heat and place under a hot grill. Cook frittata for 3 minutes or until top is set. Turn frittata on to a serving plate, and cut into wedges. Serve with 2 cups salad with low-joule dressing or balsamic vinegar or lemon juice and black pepper.

ORIENTAL PORK SALAD

<u>SERVES 4</u>

2 teaspoons sesame oil

2 tablespoons lemon juice

1 teaspoon caster sugar

2 teaspoons honey

2 teaspoons teriyaki sauce

1 clove garlic, crushed

400 g pork fillet

1 teaspoon Chinese five spice powder

cooking oil spray

150 g yellow squash, quartered

100 g snow peas, trimmed

100 g button mushrooms, sliced

1 red capsicum, chopped

100 g bean sprouts

100 g mixed lettuce leaves

In a jug, combine sesame oil, lemon juice, caster sugar, honey, teriyaki sauce and garlic, and set aside.

Spray a heated grill plate with oil. Rub pork with five spice powder and cook over medium heat, turning often, for 12–15 minutes or until tender and slightly pink in the centre. Remove pork from heat and leave to rest, covered, for 5 minutes before cutting into thin slices.

Bring a saucepan of water to the boil. Add squash and cook for 2 minutes. Add snow peas and cook for a further 30 seconds. Drain, then rinse under cold water and drain well.

In a large bowl, combine squash, snow peas, mushrooms, capsicum, bean sprouts and lettuce. Add pork, drizzle with dressing and serve.

CHAR-GRILLED TUNA WITH ROCKET CHICKPEA SALAD

SERVES 4

1 small fresh red chilli, seeded and finely chopped

1 tablespoon sweet chilli sauce

2 tablespoons lime juice

2 tablespoons fish sauce

1 tablespoon brown sugar

100 g baby rocket leaves

¼ cup fresh parsley leaves

100 g button mushrooms, thinly sliced

1 red capsicum, cut into thin strips

125 g can chickpeas, drained and rinsed

cooking oil spray

4 × 150 g tuna steaks

In a small bowl, combine chilli, sweet chilli sauce, lime juice, fish sauce and brown sugar. Stir until sugar is dissolved.

In a large bowl, combine rocket, parsley, mushrooms, capsicum and chickpeas. Cover and refrigerate for 1 hour.

Spray a heated grill plate or barbecue plate with cooking oil. Add tuna and cook until lightly browned on both sides and cooked to your liking (1–2 minutes for rare, 2–4 minutes for well done). Remove from heat, cover and set aside for a few minutes while you prepare the salad.

Remove rocket salad from refrigerator, drizzle dressing over and toss well. Arrange salad on serving plates, top with tuna and serve.

PASTA WITH FRESH TOMATO SAUCE

SERVES 4

6 medium tomatoes, peeled, seeded and coarsely chopped
½ cup coarsely chopped fresh basil, loosely packed
2 cloves garlic, crushed
2 tablespoons extra-virgin olive oil
2 teaspoons red wine vinegar
1 red Thai chilli, seeded and finely chopped
375 g fresh lasagne sheets, sliced into thick strips
80 g low-fat fetta cheese, crumbled

In a medium bowl, combine tomato, basil, garlic, half the oil, red wine vinegar and chilli.

Bring a large saucepan of salted water to the boil. Add pasta and cook, uncovered, for 10 minutes or until just tender. Remove from heat and drain. Sprinkle remaining oil over pasta, and toss gently to combine.

Arrange pasta on serving plates or in pasta bowls, spoon tomato mixture over pasta, sprinkle with cheese and serve.

SULTANA BISCUITS

<u>MAKES 40 BISCUITS</u>

1 cup self-raising flour
½ teaspoon mixed spice
40 g polyunsaturated margarine
½ cup sultanas
½ cup orange juice
½ cup rolled oats
2 tablespoons honey

Preheat oven to 180°C. Line oven trays with baking paper.

In a bowl, combine flour and mixed spice. Rub in margarine, then stir in sultanas, orange juice, oats and honey. Mix until you have a soft, wet mixture.

Spoon mixture (2 level teaspoons per biscuit) 5 cm apart on oven trays. Bake for 15 minutes or until lightly browned. Transfer biscuits to a wire rack to cool and then store in an airtight container. (Leftover biscuits can be stored in an airtight container in the freezer for up to 3 months.)

WEEK 5

Day 1

Breakfast: 1 poached egg with grilled tomato and mushrooms

Morning tea: 1 small peach

Lunch: Tuna salad: 100 grams tuna in brine or spring water, 2 cups mixed salad, 2 slices canned beetroot, 1 tablespoon toasted sesame seeds, with low-fat dressing or balsamic vinegar

Afternoon tea: 25 grams nuts

Dinner: ASIAN PORK SALAD

Supper: Low-joule jelly

Day 2

Breakfast: ⅔ cup high-fibre cereal

Morning tea: 1 small nectarine

Lunch: Chicken-and-salad sandwich: 2 slices bread, 60 grams chicken, seasoned with mustard or pickles (toast if desired)

Afternoon tea: 1 plum or 2 CHOCOLATE COOKIES

Dinner: PESTO PASTA

Supper: 1 cup strawberries

Day 3

Breakfast: 1 slice sourdough bread with 90 grams ricotta and a drizzle of honey

Morning tea: 1 small apple

Lunch: Bread roll with 45 grams rare roast beef, seeded mustard and salad

Afternoon tea: 2 fresh dates or 2 CHOCOLATE COOKIES or 30 grams (3 squares) chocolate

Dinner: CHICKEN LETTUCE CUPS

Supper: 1 icy pole (Calippo, Weiss bar) or 1 small mango

Day 4

Breakfast: 1 slice toast with 1 teaspoon peanut butter
Morning tea: 200 grams low-fat yoghurt
Lunch: 1 slice toast topped with 100 grams baked beans, served with salad
Afternoon tea: 1 scoop ice-cream or 1 icy pole or 2 apricots
Dinner: BEEF PATTIES WITH COUSCOUS
Supper: Low-joule jelly

Day 5

Breakfast: ⅔ cup cereal with 1 cup berries
Morning tea: 100 grams Fruche Lite
Lunch: Small Greek salad: salad from free list, 30 grams fetta cheese, 6 kalamata olives, with balsamic vinegar or low-joule dressing or lemon juice and black pepper
Afternoon tea: 1 small mango or 2 corn crackers with 2 tablespoons cottage cheese, tomato and black pepper
Dinner: 150 grams char-grilled salmon with mixed vegetable stir-fry
Supper: 1 plum or 2 CHOCOLATE COOKIES or 20 grams chips

Day 6

Breakfast: 1 cup fruit salad
Morning tea: 1 small pear
Lunch: 1 cheese-and-salad wrap: 1 wrap with 30 grams grated cheese and salad (toast if desired)
Afternoon tea: 15 pretzels
Dinner: SCRAMBLED EGGS WITH HERBS
Supper: 15 grapes or 30 grams (3 squares) chocolate or 1 icy pole or 1 scoop low-fat ice-cream

Day 7
Breakfast: Toasted English muffin with Vegemite or jam or honey
Morning tea: 1 small peach
Lunch: Miso soup, 2 sushi rolls
Afternoon tea: 10 cherries or 2 CHOCOLATE COOKIES
Dinner: VEAL WITH ONIONS served with 2 cups salad or stir-fried vegetables
Supper: 1 cup rhubarb with 1 tablespoon low-fat custard

Recipes for Week 5

ASIAN PORK SALAD

<u>SERVES 4</u>

1/3 cup fat-free honey soy dressing
1 tablespoon lime juice
1 clove garlic, crushed
1 small fresh red chilli, finely chopped
cooking oil spray
500 g pork fillet
1/4 red cabbage, finely shredded
1 medium green capsicum, thinly sliced
1 small carrot, grated
1/3 cup roughly chopped flat-leafed parsley
1/3 cup chopped fresh mint leaves
4 spring onions, thinly sliced

In a jar with a screw-top lid, combine honey soy dressing, lime juice, garlic and chilli. Tighten lid and shake well.

Spray a large heated non-stick frying pan with oil. Add pork and cook over medium heat for 15–17 minutes, turning frequently, until browned all over and slightly pink in the centre. Remove from heat and leave to rest for 5 minutes before cutting into thin slices.

In a large bowl, combine cabbage, capsicum, carrot, parsley, mint leaves and spring onion. Add pork and dressing, toss salad and serve.

PESTO PASTA

<u>SERVES 4</u>

2 cups basil leaves, firmly packed

1 clove garlic

1 tablespoon toasted pine nuts

1 tablespoon grated Parmesan cheese

1/4 cup fat-free herb-and-garlic salad dressing

375 g packet fresh cheese-and-tomato ravioli

250 g punnet cherry tomatoes, halved

4 spring onions, finely chopped

salt and pepper, to taste

In the bowl of an electric blender, combine basil, garlic, pine nuts, cheese and dressing. Blend until mixture is pureed.

Bring a large saucepan of salted water to the boil. Add pasta and cook, uncovered, for 6 minutes or until tender. Remove from heat and drain, then rinse under cold water and drain well.

In a large bowl, combine pasta, tomatoes and spring onions. Add pesto, season with salt and pepper, mix well and serve.

CHICKEN LETTUCE CUPS

<u>SERVES 4</u>

4 large iceberg lettuce leaves
1 tablespoon teriyaki sauce
1 teaspoon sesame oil
125 g chicken breast fillet
1 large carrot, coarsely grated
2 sticks celery, finely sliced
4 spring onions, finely sliced
2 tablespoons sweet chilli sauce

With scissors, trim the edges of the lettuce leaves to form cups. Place leaves in a large bowl of iced water, then cover and refrigerate overnight.

In a bowl, combine teriyaki sauce and sesame oil. Add chicken and mix well to thoroughly coat chicken with marinade. Leave to rest for 15 minutes. Drain chicken and then pat dry on absorbent paper.

Heat a non-stick frying pan. Add chicken and cook for 3 minutes on each side or until browned and cooked through. Remove chicken from heat and leave to rest for 5 minutes before cutting into thin slices.

In a large bowl, combine chicken, carrot, celery, spring onions and chilli sauce. Mix well.

Drain lettuce leaves, dry well and arrange on four serving plates. Spoon chicken mixture into lettuce cups and serve.

BEEF PATTIES WITH COUSCOUS
SERVES 4

400 g lean minced beef
1 small onion, finely chopped
1 clove garlic, crushed
2 teaspoons dried mixed herbs
cooking oil spray
¾ cup couscous
¾ cup boiling water
1 teaspoon finely grated lemon rind
2 tablespoons lemon juice
¼ cup chopped fresh parsley
½ cup low-fat plain yoghurt, to serve

In a large bowl, combine beef, onion, garlic and herbs. With your hands, mix well. With wet hands, divide mixture into four portions and shape into patties. Cover and refrigerate for 30 minutes.

Spray a heated grill plate with oil. Cook patties for 3 minutes on each side or until browned and cooked through.

While patties are cooking, combine couscous, boiling water and lemon rind in a heatproof bowl. Cover and leave to rest for 5 minutes. With a fork, fluff couscous, then stir in lemon juice and parsley.

Arrange couscous on serving plates and place patties on top. Drizzle yoghurt over and serve.

SCRAMBLED EGGS WITH HERBS
SERVES 4

8 eggs
¾ cup reduced-fat milk
¼ cup finely chopped fresh parsley
salt and pepper, to taste
2 large tomatoes, halved
1 tablespoon dried breadcrumbs
1 tablespoon grated Parmesan cheese
1 clove garlic, crushed
1 tablespoon chopped fresh parsley
cooking oil spray
100 g packet baby spinach leaves

In a jug, combine eggs, milk and parsley, and season with salt and pepper. Whisk until combined.

On an oven tray, arrange tomatoes cut-side down. Cook under a hot grill for 3–4 minutes or until skins start to blister.

Meanwhile, combine breadcrumbs, cheese, garlic and parsley in a bowl. Remove tomatoes from heat and turn over. Sprinkle with breadcrumb mixture and spray with a little oil. Return tomatoes to grill and cook until crumbs are toasted.

As tomatoes are grilling, heat a large non-stick frying pan. Add egg mixture and cook over medium heat, stirring occasionally with a wooden spoon, for 5 minutes or until eggs are almost set. Stir in the spinach.

Serve scrambled eggs with tomatoes.

VEAL WITH ONIONS
SERVES 4

2 tablespoons lemon juice
1 teaspoon grain mustard
1 teaspoon paprika
1 clove garlic, crushed
4 × 125 g veal leg steaks
1 teaspoon olive oil
4 white onions, thinly sliced
1 tablespoon chopped fresh thyme
salt and pepper, to taste

In a bowl, combine lemon juice, mustard, paprika and garlic. Add veal and mix well to thoroughly coat veal with marinade. Cover and leave to rest for 15 minutes.

Heat oil in a large non-stick frying pan. Add onions and thyme, and season with salt and pepper. Cook, stirring, over low heat for 20 minutes or until soft and golden brown. Transfer onions to a plate and keep pan over heat.

Drain veal, reserving marinade in a bowl. Add veal to heated pan and cook for 2 minutes on each side or until tender. Arrange veal on serving plates. Return onions to frying pan and scrape in reserved marinade. Increase heat and bring to boil, stirring, for 30 seconds. Pour onions over veal, and serve with 2 cups salad or 2 cups stir-fried vegetables.

CHOCOLATE COOKIES
MAKES 48 COOKIES

⅓ cup cocoa powder

1½ cups plain flour

½ teaspoon baking powder

185 g unsalted butter, softened

½ cup caster sugar

2 egg yolks

2 tablespoons white chocolate bits

Preheat oven to 160°C. Line oven trays with baking paper.

Sift cocoa powder, flour and baking powder together.

In the bowl of an electric mixer, combine butter, sugar and egg yolks. Mix until just combined, then stir in cocoa mixture and mix well.

Roll mixture into balls (2 teaspoons per cookie) and place 4 cm apart on oven trays. Press a chocolate bit into the centre of each cookie.

Bake for 12–15 minutes or until cookies are cooked through. Remove from oven and allow to cool on trays. Store cookies in an airtight container. (Leftover cookies can be stored in an airtight container in the freezer for up to 3 months.)

WEEK 6

Day 1
Breakfast: 1 cup strawberries with 200 grams low-fat yoghurt
Morning tea: 1 small orange
Lunch: Turkey sandwich: 2 slices wholegrain bread, 60 grams turkey breast and salad, flavoured with cranberry jelly if desired
Afternoon tea: 2 COCONUT COOKIES or 2 plain biscuits
Dinner: TOMATO OLIVE PASTA
Supper: 1 Jarrah hot chocolate or Swiss Miss or Cadbury Lite or Ovaltine Lite

Day 2
Breakfast: 2 Weetbix
Morning tea: 1 small mandarin
Lunch: Tuna-and-salad sandwich: 2 slices wholegrain or rye bread, 100 grams canned tuna, 2 teaspoons low-fat mayonnaise
Afternoon tea: 1 small pear
Dinner: FISH FILLETS WITH BASIL SAUCE served with 2 cups salad
Supper: 100 grams Fruche Lite

Day 3
Breakfast: 1 egg (poached or scrambled) with grilled tomato and mushrooms
Morning tea: 1 tangello
Lunch: Cheese-and-salad wrap: 1 wrap with 30 grams tasty cheese, tomato, lettuce, cucumber, capsicum and canned beetroot (toast if desired)
Afternoon tea: 25 grams nuts and raisins
Dinner: CHICKEN COTTAGE PIES served with 2 cups salad or 2 cups steamed vegetables
Supper: Low-joule jelly

Day 4
Breakfast: 1 slice crusty bread with 3 cherry tomatoes (halved) and 2 tablespoons ricotta, all melted and seasoned with cracked black pepper
Morning tea: 1 small apple
Lunch: QUICK NICOISE SALAD
Afternoon tea: 1 corn cob
Dinner: SPICY PUMPKIN SOUP
Supper: 1 Jarrah hot chocolate or Swiss Miss or Cadbury Lite or Ovaltine Lite

Day 5
Breakfast: ⅔ cup high-fibre cereal
Morning tea: 125 grams canned fruit
Lunch: Bagel with 2 slices smoked salmon and salad
Afternoon tea: 1 cup 98% fat-free soup (Continental, Country Cup)
Dinner: BEEF WITH OYSTER SAUCE
Supper: 2 COCONUT COOKIES or 30 grams (3 squares) chocolate

Day 6
Breakfast: 2-egg omelette with tomato, mushrooms, capsicum
Morning tea: 10 cherries
Lunch: SPICY PUMPKIN SOUP
Afternoon tea: 1 small slice chocolate cake/tangello
Dinner: 150 grams grilled fish with 2 cups vegetables or salad
Supper: 1 cup rhubarb with 2 tablespoons low-fat custard

Day 7

Breakfast: ½ cup porridge

Morning tea: 1 cup cubed watermelon

Lunch: Miso soup, 2 sushi rolls

Afternoon tea: 2 COCONUT COOKIES or 1 chocolate biscuit

Dinner: MARINATED CHILLI LIME LAMB served with 2 cups steamed vegetables

Supper: 1 cup berries

Recipes for Week 6

TOMATO OLIVE PASTA
SERVES 4

250 g spiral pasta
2 × 410 g cans chopped tomatoes
1 teaspoon dried Italian herbs
½ cup black olives, sliced
½ × 56 g can anchovy fillets, finely chopped
2 teaspoons baby capers, drained
2 tablespoons chopped fresh basil

Bring a saucepan of salted water to the boil. Add pasta and cook uncovered for 10 minutes or until just tender. Remove from heat and drain.

While pasta is cooking, place tomatoes and dried herbs in a saucepan. Bring to boil and then reduce heat and simmer, uncovered, for 6–7 minutes or until mixture thickens. Stir in olives, anchovies, capers and basil. Pour sauce over pasta and toss well. Arrange pasta in four pasta bowls and serve.

FISH FILLETS WITH BASIL SAUCE
SERVES 4

⅓ cup low-fat mayonnaise

1 tablespoon basil pesto

2 teaspoons lemon juice

½ teaspoon paprika

½ teaspoon ground cumin

½ teaspoon salt

4 × 150 g boneless fish fillets

cooking oil spray

In a small jug, combine mayonnaise, pesto and lemon juice. Mix well.

In a small bowl, combine paprika, cumin and salt. Line an oven tray with foil and place fish fillets on foil. Spray one side of each fillet with a little oil, then sprinkle spice mixture evenly over top.

Cook fish fillets (don't turn them over) under a hot grill for 7–8 minutes or until browned and cooked through.

Arrange fish on serving plates, drizzle basil sauce over fish and serve with 2 cups salad.

CHICKEN COTTAGE PIES

<u>SERVES 4</u>

4 medium potatoes, peeled and coarsely chopped
¼ cup reduced-fat milk
salt and pepper, to taste
cooking oil spray
400 g minced chicken
1 small onion, finely chopped
2 sticks celery, finely chopped
1 carrot, finely chopped
1 tablespoon Worcestershire sauce
400 g can chopped tomatoes
½ cup water
250 g packet frozen spinach, thawed and chopped

Preheat oven to 200°C. Grease four (1¼-cup capacity) ovenproof dishes and place on an oven tray.

Bring a large saucepan of salted water to a simmer. Add potatoes and simmer, uncovered, for 20 minutes or until tender. Remove from heat and drain, then return potatoes to saucepan and add milk. Mash until smooth, then season with salt and pepper. Cover to keep warm.

Spray a large heated frying pan with oil. Add chicken, onion, celery and carrot, and cook, stirring, for 5 minutes or until chicken is white. Add Worcestershire sauce, tomatoes and water. Increase heat and bring to the boil, then reduce heat and simmer, stirring occasionally, for 10 minutes or until thickened.

Squeeze moisture from spinach and then stir into chicken mixture. Divide mixture among prepared dishes, then top with mashed potato.

Bake for 20 minutes or until tops are browned. Serve the pies in their oven dishes.

QUICK NICOISE SALAD

<u>SERVES 4</u>

3 cups thin French green beans
4 large Desiree potatoes, thinly sliced
½ teaspoon salt
200 g bottle roasted capsicum, rinsed and thinly sliced
cracked black pepper, to taste
400 g canned tuna in brine, lightly drained and flaked
12 kalamata olives, drained
4 teaspoons white wine vinegar

Place beans in a large bowl.

Bring a saucepan of salted water to the boil. Add potatoes and cook for 5 minutes or until tender. Remove from heat and drain through sieve over the beans, and leave both to rest for 5 minutes.

Drain beans, then add potatoes, capsicum and ½ teaspoon salt, and season with black pepper.

Toss salad and arrange on four serving plates. Divide tuna and olives between the salads, sprinkle each with 1 teaspoon vinegar and serve.

SPICY PUMPKIN SOUP

<u>SERVES 4</u>

2 teaspoons olive oil

1 small onion, chopped

2 cloves garlic, crushed

2 teaspoons ground cumin

½ teaspoon ground turmeric

250 g sweet potato, peeled and chopped

500 g pumpkin, peeled and chopped

3 cups chicken stock

½ cup lite coconut cream

salt and pepper, to taste

2 tablespoons chopped fresh chives, to serve

Heat oil in a large saucepan. Add onion, garlic and spices and cook, stirring, for 2–3 minutes or until soft. Add sweet potato, pumpkin and stock. Increase heat and bring to boil, then reduce heat and simmer, covered, for 20 minutes or until tender. Remove from heat and allow to cool slightly.

In an electric mixer, blend soup in batches until smooth. Return soup to pan and stir in coconut milk over heat until hot. Season with salt and pepper and sprinkle with chives. Pour soup into soup bowls and serve.

BEEF WITH OYSTER SAUCE

<u>SERVES 4</u>

1 tablespoon dark soy sauce

1 tablespoon dry sherry

1 clove garlic, crushed

500 g beef strips

½ cup beef stock

2 teaspoons cornflour

2 teaspoons peanut oil

1 medium onion, cut into wedges

2 bunches (6 stalks) broccolini, chopped

2 yellow zucchini, sliced

1 medium carrot, thinly sliced

100 g snow peas, trimmed

2 tablespoons oyster sauce

In a bowl, combine soy sauce, sherry and garlic. Add beef and mix well to thoroughly coat beef with marinade. Cover and refrigerate for 30 minutes.

In a separate bowl, blend stock and cornflour.

Heat oil in a wok or non-stick frying pan. Add beef, in batches (cooking in batches will brown the meat rather than stew it) and stir-fry for 2–3 minutes or until browned all over. Remove from wok and set aside on a warm plate.

Add onion, broccolini, zucchini and carrot to wok, and stir-fry for 3 minutes or until vegetables are just tender. Return beef to wok and add snow peas, oyster sauce and stock and cornflour mixture. Stir-fry until mixture boils and thickens and then serve.

MARINATED CHILLI LIME LAMB

<u>SERVES 4</u>

cooking oil spray
500 g lamb fillets
2 teaspoons grated lemon rind
½ cup palm sugar
2 tablespoons lime juice
2 tablespoons water
1 fresh red chilli, seeded and finely chopped
1 tablespoon chopped fresh coriander

Spray a heated grill plate with oil. Add lamb fillets and cook for 3–4 minutes, turning frequently, or until tender on both sides. Remove lamb from heat and slice.

While lamb is cooking, combine sugar, lime juice and water in a small saucepan. Stir over heat, without boiling, for 3 minutes or until sugar has dissolved. Simmer, uncovered, without stirring for 2 minutes, then remove from heat to cool slightly. Stir in chilli and coriander.

Arrange lamb slices on serving plates, drizzle over chilli sauce and serve with 2 cups steamed vegetables.

COCONUT COOKIES

<u>MAKES 50 COOKIES</u>

185 g butter, softened
½ cup brown sugar, firmly packed
1 egg
1 teaspoon vanilla extract
1¼ cups self-raising flour, sifted
½ cup plain flour, sifted
½ cup desiccated coconut

Preheat oven to 180°C. Lightly grease oven trays.

In the bowl of an electric mixer, combine butter and sugar. Mix until light and fluffy, then add egg and vanilla, and mix well. Add sifted flours and coconut, and mix well until you have a soft dough.

Roll teaspoonfuls of mixture into balls and place on oven trays. With a fork, lightly flatten each ball.

Bake for 10 minutes or until golden brown. Remove from oven and cool on a wire rack. Store cookies in an airtight container. (Leftover cookies can be stored in an airtight container in the freezer for up to 3 months.)

CHAPTER 17

Tips for eating out and takeaway – the healthy way

There is a sensible approach to eating out and ordering take-away food. Your new lifestyle allows you to try an assortment of restaurants to see which you enjoy – all are adaptable to your new eating plan. Here are some simple guidelines about names of dishes, cooking methods, common ingredients and the most appropriate dishes for a wide variety of dine-in or takeaway restaurants. These will assist you in making the right choices.

1. Do not be shy to ask your waiter about the ingredients and cooking methods of dishes with which you are not familiar.

2. Do not hesitate to ask for specially prepared meals or alterations to standard menu items. Most restaurants will be obliging. Remember, you are paying!

3. Ask for an entree-size meal instead of a main-course portion. If you are ordering two courses, order two entrees instead of an entree and a main meal.

4. When an item on the menu *really* appeals to you, but it

has a rich buttery sauce or an oily dressing, order it with the sauce or the dressing on the side.

5. Order extra steamed vegetables, but stipulate you want them without butter.

6. If you feel like something sweet, try a spoonful of someone else's dessert; this way you still get to sample the delicious taste.

7. Don't worry about leaving food on your plate. When you are comfortably full stop eating and ask the waiter to take the leftovers away before you nibble at them.

8. Eat slowly and talk a lot.

9. Have a glass of water before and between each glass of wine.

Bon appetit!

Below is some advice on how to select meals from a range of wonderful cuisines. Remember, variety is the spice of life!

THAI, VIETNAMESE AND MALAYSIAN

- Clear soups with added meat and vegetables are excellent, delicious and filling choices.
- Choose meat or vegetarian dishes served in chilli-based spicy sauce instead of satay sauce.
- Avoid all dishes with added coconut/coconut milk.
- Try hot or cold salad dishes such as Thai Beef Salad.
- A vegetable stir-fry with chicken, fish or lean meat is a tasty choice.

- Select steamed rice or noodles as an accompaniment to your meal. Be aware that ⅓ cup of rice/pasta/noodles = 1 carbohydrate serve.
- Avoid fried rice and noodle dishes such as Mee Grob.
- Healthy choices include Thai Beef Salad, Hot Sour Prawn Soup, Tom Yum Goong, Tom Yum Phak, Chilli Prawns, Fish in Tamarind Sauce, Thai Green Mango Salad and Mixed Seafood with Basil.

MEXICAN

- Beware! Most dishes contain liberal amounts of sour cream, avocado and cheese, so choose carefully. Ask the waiter to omit these from your dish (or use sparingly).
- Frijoles (bean) or Verocruz (tomato) dips with a few corn chips are a tasty way to begin the meal. A Fiesta Salad with the dressing on the side is a good alternative.
- Choose soft tortillas such as Enchiladas and Burritos instead of fried tortillas like Tostada and Quesadilla. Fill with salad, fish, lean meat, chicken or beans.
- Check other dishes on the menu, you may find a suitable meat dish served in a spicy Mexican sauce.

LOCAL CLUB/HOTEL

- Grilled fish of the day served with salad or vegetables is a good choice.
- Ask for a small serve of grilled meat or share a steak between two people.
- Request that your meal be served with boiled or jacket

potatoes instead of chips, or perhaps some boiled rice or pasta. Remember portion sizes!

- Dessert selections usually include fruit salad or sorbet, or finish the meal with a cup of one of the numerous teas now available, or a well brewed cup of coffee.

JAPANESE

Japanese food is usually fresh, light and very healthy. There are, however, a few hidden traps so use the following ideas as a guide.

- Miso soup as an entree is a traditional starter, and takes the edge off your appetite.
- Sashimi (raw seafood) and sushi (seafood with rice) are great as meal starters or as main meals accompanied by ginger or wasabi to add a bit of spice.
- Good choices are teriyaki (marinated meat), Yakitore (chicken kebabs) and Yosenabe (poached seafood and raw vegetables). They are preferable to Sukiyake (meat with raw egg) and Tempura (assorted fried items).
- Choose noodles (Udon, Soba) that are steamed or in broth, not fried.
- Fried eggplant, fried tofu and egg dishes are best avoided. Choose marinated tofu or eggplant dishes instead.
- Dessert items often contain coconut and are best avoided.

CHINESE

- Choose clear soups; chicken-and-corn is very satisfying – often sufficient for a meal.

- Avoid creamy or egg-based soups.
- Choose steamed rice or noodles rather than fried varieties. Be aware that ⅓ cup of rice/pasta/noodles = 1 carbohydrate serve.
- Try combined meat and vegetable dishes rather than those with meat alone. (Select fish and chicken dishes prepared without fat.)
- Vegetarian dishes are a good idea – try Vegetables in Oyster Sauce, Vegetables in Black Bean Sauce, stir-fried vegetables or steamed vegetables.
- Avoid duck and deep-fried or battered dishes.
- Limit or avoid dishes containing nuts or seeds, because they increase the fat content of the dish.
- Ask for steamed spring rolls and dim sims.
- Sweet-and-sour dishes tend to be high in fat, as are omelettes and satay dishes.

ITALIAN
- Minestrone or lentil-based soups are excellent entree choices, but try and omit the Parmesan; for flavour, use cracked black pepper instead.
- A salad is a good alternative for a starter, with the dressing on the side.
- Choose a tomato-based pasta sauce such as Napolitana with seafood, lean meat or vegetables. Forget the Pesto, Lasagna, Cannelloni and cheesy sauces.
- Be careful with the quantity of pasta/rice/gnocchi you consume; remember that ⅓ cup = 1 carbohydrate serve.

- Chicken, seafood or veal dishes served with vegetables or salad are acceptable choices if the meat is grilled or prepared in a tomato-based casserole.
- Avoid ice-cream – a refreshing fruity gelato is a delicious full stop to the meal.
- For tips on pizza, see the pizza section on page 298.

LEBANESE

- Most vegetarian dishes – such as hummus and tahini – are acceptable.
- Choose lean meat dishes such as shish kebabs, shwarma, souvlaki and cabbage rolls.
- Avoid egg-based dishes such as omelettes.
- Tabouli and Lebanese bread are excellent accompaniments to a meal.
- Avoid baklava and similar pastry desserts.
- Falafel is deep-fried in oil so it is best avoided.

INDIAN

- Omit all dishes with coconut milk.
- Mulligatawny soup is a tasty, low-fat meal starter.
- Try the authentic Tandoori oven dishes – rice and vegetables with fish, chicken, seafood or lamb.
- Chicken Tikka is a delicious starter or main course.
- Biriyani and Vindaloo dishes are much lower in fat than Korma curry, so they make a better choice.
- Try to include a vegetable dish instead of having only meat dishes.

- Dahl (lentils) and Raita (yoghurt and dip) are pleasant meal accompaniments.
- Avoid fried entree items such as Pakoras and Samosas.
- Select baked breads (Naan, Roti, Chappati) rather than fried bread (Pappadums, Parathas, Puri) – request the chef not to add butter.
- Cool Indian drinks such as Sharbat (fruity) and Lhassi (yoghurt based) are excellent thirst quenchers, and a good alternative to alcohol.

KFC

- Remove both batter and skin from the chicken. Select the breast rather than the wing or drumstick.
- Choose corn on the cob, mashed potato and gravy, bean salad and coleslaw instead of fried chips.

PIZZA

- Avoid deep-pan pizzas that are laden with fat.
- Select pizzas with a crusty dough base topped with plenty of vegetables, such as capsicum, mushrooms, onions, pineapple, olives and tomatoes. Steer clear of salami, bacon, cabanossi, pepperoni and extra cheese. Choose lean ham, prawns and other seafood.
- Make use of the salad bar but avoid salads with a lot of high-fat dressing.
- Select pasta dishes as indicated for Italian restaurants (see page 296).

McDONALD'S

- Breakfast at the golden arches offers a variety of cereals, English muffins and fruit.
- Garden or chicken salad with low-fat French, Italian or mango-and-sesame dressings are healthy options.
- A lean beef burger or chicken foldover are good choices.

CHICKEN SHOPS

- Ask for a char-grilled burger without the mayonnaise or enjoy a grilled chicken salad.
- Chicken breast in pita without mayonnaise is a good alternative.
- If you order rice, remember that ⅓ cup = 1 carbohydrate serve.
- Chicken breast (remove the skin and stuffing) with salad is an excellent selection.
- Salads are great, but be wary of the dressings.

EATING AT A FRIEND'S HOUSE

- Have a low-fat snack such as a soup, salad or yoghurt before you leave home to keep you going until dinner is served.
- Avoid the appetisers that are passed around with drinks.
- Start with a mineral water, diet drink or soda water and only move on to wine with your meal.
- Top your wine glass with water to prevent it being constantly refilled.
- Ignore the bread.

- Don't feel obliged to finish everything on your plate.
- When dessert is offered, ask for a small portion to taste.
- Feel confident to remark on the delicious meal, but if you are full tell your host that you have had enough to eat.

Index